Weekly Diabetes Record

Name: _____

Date:	Breakfast	Snack	Lunch	Snack	Dinner	Snack	Bedtime	Night	Notes
Blood Sugar									
Insulin Dose									
Grams Carb									
Activity									

Date:	Breakfast	Snack	Lunch	Snack	Dinner	Snack	Bedtime	Night	Notes
Blood Sugar									
Insulin Dose									
Grams Carb									
Activity									

Date:	Breakfast	Snack	Lunch	Snack	Dinner	Snack	Bedtime	Night	Notes
Blood Sugar									
Insulin Dose									
Grams Carb									
Activity									

Date:	Breakfast	Snack	Lunch	Snack	Dinner	Snack	Bedtime	Night	Notes
Blood Sugar									
Insulin Dose									
Grams Carb									
Activity									

Date:	Breakfast	Snack	Lunch	Snack	Dinner	Snack	Bedtime	Night	Notes
Blood Sugar									
Insulin Dose									
Grams Carb									
Activity									

Date:	Breakfast	Snack	Lunch	Snack	Dinner	Snack	Bedtime	Night	Notes
Blood Sugar									
Insulin Dose									
Grams Carb									
Activity									

Date:	Breakfast	Snack	Lunch	Snack	Dinner	Snack	Bedtime	Night	Notes
Blood Sugar									
Insulin Dose									
Grams Carb									
Activity									

Weekly Diabetes Record

Name: _____

Date:	Breakfast	Snack	Lunch	Snack	Dinner	Snack	Bedtime	Night	Notes
Blood Sugar									
Insulin Dose									
Grams Carb									
Activity									

Date:	Breakfast	Snack	Lunch	Snack	Dinner	Snack	Bedtime	Night	Notes
Blood Sugar									
Insulin Dose									
Grams Carb									
Activity									

Date:	Breakfast	Snack	Lunch	Snack	Dinner	Snack	Bedtime	Night	Notes
Blood Sugar									
Insulin Dose									
Grams Carb									
Activity									

Date:	Breakfast	Snack	Lunch	Snack	Dinner	Snack	Bedtime	Night	Notes
Blood Sugar									
Insulin Dose									
Grams Carb									
Activity									

Date:	Breakfast	Snack	Lunch	Snack	Dinner	Snack	Bedtime	Night	Notes
Blood Sugar									
Insulin Dose									
Grams Carb									
Activity									

Date:	Breakfast	Snack	Lunch	Snack	Dinner	Snack	Bedtime	Night	Notes
Blood Sugar									
Insulin Dose									
Grams Carb									
Activity									

Date:	Breakfast	Snack	Lunch	Snack	Dinner	Snack	Bedtime	Night	Notes
Blood Sugar									
Insulin Dose									
Grams Carb									
Activity									

Weekly Diabetes Record

Name: _____

Date:	Breakfast	Snack	Lunch	Snack	Dinner	Snack	Bedtime	Night	Notes
Blood Sugar									
Insulin Dose									
Grams Carb									
Activity									

Date:	Breakfast	Snack	Lunch	Snack	Dinner	Snack	Bedtime	Night	Notes
Blood Sugar									
Insulin Dose									
Grams Carb									
Activity									

Date:	Breakfast	Snack	Lunch	Snack	Dinner	Snack	Bedtime	Night	Notes
Blood Sugar									
Insulin Dose									
Grams Carb									
Activity									

Date:	Breakfast	Snack	Lunch	Snack	Dinner	Snack	Bedtime	Night	Notes
Blood Sugar									
Insulin Dose									
Grams Carb									
Activity									

Date:	Breakfast	Snack	Lunch	Snack	Dinner	Snack	Bedtime	Night	Notes
Blood Sugar									
Insulin Dose									
Grams Carb									
Activity									

Date:	Breakfast	Snack	Lunch	Snack	Dinner	Snack	Bedtime	Night	Notes
Blood Sugar									
Insulin Dose									
Grams Carb									
Activity									

Date:	Breakfast	Snack	Lunch	Snack	Dinner	Snack	Bedtime	Night	Notes
Blood Sugar									
Insulin Dose									
Grams Carb									
Activity									

Weekly Diabetes Record

Name: _____

Date:	Breakfast	Snack	Lunch	Snack	Dinner	Snack	Bedtime	Night	Notes
Blood Sugar									
Insulin Dose									
Grams Carb									
Activity									

Date:	Breakfast	Snack	Lunch	Snack	Dinner	Snack	Bedtime	Night	Notes
Blood Sugar									
Insulin Dose									
Grams Carb									
Activity									

Date:	Breakfast	Snack	Lunch	Snack	Dinner	Snack	Bedtime	Night	Notes
Blood Sugar									
Insulin Dose									
Grams Carb									
Activity									

Date:	Breakfast	Snack	Lunch	Snack	Dinner	Snack	Bedtime	Night	Notes
Blood Sugar									
Insulin Dose									
Grams Carb									
Activity									

Date:	Breakfast	Snack	Lunch	Snack	Dinner	Snack	Bedtime	Night	Notes
Blood Sugar									
Insulin Dose									
Grams Carb									
Activity									

Date:	Breakfast	Snack	Lunch	Snack	Dinner	Snack	Bedtime	Night	Notes
Blood Sugar									
Insulin Dose									
Grams Carb									
Activity									

Date:	Breakfast	Snack	Lunch	Snack	Dinner	Snack	Bedtime	Night	Notes
Blood Sugar									
Insulin Dose									
Grams Carb									
Activity									

Weekly Diabetes Record

Name: _____

Date:	Breakfast	Snack	Lunch	Snack	Dinner	Snack	Bedtime	Night	Notes
Blood Sugar									
Insulin Dose									
Grams Carb									
Activity									

Date:	Breakfast	Snack	Lunch	Snack	Dinner	Snack	Bedtime	Night	Notes
Blood Sugar									
Insulin Dose									
Grams Carb									
Activity									

Date:	Breakfast	Snack	Lunch	Snack	Dinner	Snack	Bedtime	Night	Notes
Blood Sugar									
Insulin Dose									
Grams Carb									
Activity									

Date:	Breakfast	Snack	Lunch	Snack	Dinner	Snack	Bedtime	Night	Notes
Blood Sugar									
Insulin Dose									
Grams Carb									
Activity									

Date:	Breakfast	Snack	Lunch	Snack	Dinner	Snack	Bedtime	Night	Notes
Blood Sugar									
Insulin Dose									
Grams Carb									
Activity									

Date:	Breakfast	Snack	Lunch	Snack	Dinner	Snack	Bedtime	Night	Notes
Blood Sugar									
Insulin Dose									
Grams Carb									
Activity									

Date:	Breakfast	Snack	Lunch	Snack	Dinner	Snack	Bedtime	Night	Notes
Blood Sugar									
Insulin Dose									
Grams Carb									
Activity									

Weekly Diabetes Record

Name: _____

Date:	Breakfast	Snack	Lunch	Snack	Dinner	Snack	Bedtime	Night	Notes
Blood Sugar									
Insulin Dose									
Grams Carb									
Activity									

Date:	Breakfast	Snack	Lunch	Snack	Dinner	Snack	Bedtime	Night	Notes
Blood Sugar									
Insulin Dose									
Grams Carb									
Activity									

Date:	Breakfast	Snack	Lunch	Snack	Dinner	Snack	Bedtime	Night	Notes
Blood Sugar									
Insulin Dose									
Grams Carb									
Activity									

Date:	Breakfast	Snack	Lunch	Snack	Dinner	Snack	Bedtime	Night	Notes
Blood Sugar									
Insulin Dose									
Grams Carb									
Activity									

Date:	Breakfast	Snack	Lunch	Snack	Dinner	Snack	Bedtime	Night	Notes
Blood Sugar									
Insulin Dose									
Grams Carb									
Activity									

Date:	Breakfast	Snack	Lunch	Snack	Dinner	Snack	Bedtime	Night	Notes
Blood Sugar									
Insulin Dose									
Grams Carb									
Activity									

Date:	Breakfast	Snack	Lunch	Snack	Dinner	Snack	Bedtime	Night	Notes
Blood Sugar									
Insulin Dose									
Grams Carb									
Activity									

Weekly Diabetes Record

Name: _____

Date:	Breakfast	Snack	Lunch	Snack	Dinner	Snack	Bedtime	Night	Notes
Blood Sugar									
Insulin Dose									
Grams Carb									
Activity									

Date:	Breakfast	Snack	Lunch	Snack	Dinner	Snack	Bedtime	Night	Notes
Blood Sugar									
Insulin Dose									
Grams Carb									
Activity									

Date:	Breakfast	Snack	Lunch	Snack	Dinner	Snack	Bedtime	Night	Notes
Blood Sugar									
Insulin Dose									
Grams Carb									
Activity									

Date:	Breakfast	Snack	Lunch	Snack	Dinner	Snack	Bedtime	Night	Notes
Blood Sugar									
Insulin Dose									
Grams Carb									
Activity									

Date:	Breakfast	Snack	Lunch	Snack	Dinner	Snack	Bedtime	Night	Notes
Blood Sugar									
Insulin Dose									
Grams Carb									
Activity									

Date:	Breakfast	Snack	Lunch	Snack	Dinner	Snack	Bedtime	Night	Notes
Blood Sugar									
Insulin Dose									
Grams Carb									
Activity									

Date:	Breakfast	Snack	Lunch	Snack	Dinner	Snack	Bedtime	Night	Notes
Blood Sugar									
Insulin Dose									
Grams Carb									
Activity									

Weekly Diabetes Record

Name: _____

Date:	Breakfast	Snack	Lunch	Snack	Dinner	Snack	Bedtime	Night	Notes
Blood Sugar									
Insulin Dose									
Grams Carb									
Activity									

Date:	Breakfast	Snack	Lunch	Snack	Dinner	Snack	Bedtime	Night	Notes
Blood Sugar									
Insulin Dose									
Grams Carb									
Activity									

Date:	Breakfast	Snack	Lunch	Snack	Dinner	Snack	Bedtime	Night	Notes
Blood Sugar									
Insulin Dose									
Grams Carb									
Activity									

Date:	Breakfast	Snack	Lunch	Snack	Dinner	Snack	Bedtime	Night	Notes
Blood Sugar									
Insulin Dose									
Grams Carb									
Activity									

Date:	Breakfast	Snack	Lunch	Snack	Dinner	Snack	Bedtime	Night	Notes
Blood Sugar									
Insulin Dose									
Grams Carb									
Activity									

Date:	Breakfast	Snack	Lunch	Snack	Dinner	Snack	Bedtime	Night	Notes
Blood Sugar									
Insulin Dose									
Grams Carb									
Activity									

Date:	Breakfast	Snack	Lunch	Snack	Dinner	Snack	Bedtime	Night	Notes
Blood Sugar									
Insulin Dose									
Grams Carb									
Activity									

Weekly Diabetes Record

Name: _____

Date:	Breakfast	Snack	Lunch	Snack	Dinner	Snack	Bedtime	Night	Notes
Blood Sugar									
Insulin Dose									
Grams Carb									
Activity									

Date:	Breakfast	Snack	Lunch	Snack	Dinner	Snack	Bedtime	Night	Notes
Blood Sugar									
Insulin Dose									
Grams Carb									
Activity									

Date:	Breakfast	Snack	Lunch	Snack	Dinner	Snack	Bedtime	Night	Notes
Blood Sugar									
Insulin Dose									
Grams Carb									
Activity									

Date:	Breakfast	Snack	Lunch	Snack	Dinner	Snack	Bedtime	Night	Notes
Blood Sugar									
Insulin Dose									
Grams Carb									
Activity									

Date:	Breakfast	Snack	Lunch	Snack	Dinner	Snack	Bedtime	Night	Notes
Blood Sugar									
Insulin Dose									
Grams Carb									
Activity									

Date:	Breakfast	Snack	Lunch	Snack	Dinner	Snack	Bedtime	Night	Notes
Blood Sugar									
Insulin Dose									
Grams Carb									
Activity									

Date:	Breakfast	Snack	Lunch	Snack	Dinner	Snack	Bedtime	Night	Notes
Blood Sugar									
Insulin Dose									
Grams Carb									
Activity									

Weekly Diabetes Record

Name: _____

Date:	Breakfast	Snack	Lunch	Snack	Dinner	Snack	Bedtime	Night	Notes
Blood Sugar									
Insulin Dose									
Grams Carb									
Activity									

Date:	Breakfast	Snack	Lunch	Snack	Dinner	Snack	Bedtime	Night	Notes
Blood Sugar									
Insulin Dose									
Grams Carb									
Activity									

Date:	Breakfast	Snack	Lunch	Snack	Dinner	Snack	Bedtime	Night	Notes
Blood Sugar									
Insulin Dose									
Grams Carb									
Activity									

Date:	Breakfast	Snack	Lunch	Snack	Dinner	Snack	Bedtime	Night	Notes
Blood Sugar									
Insulin Dose									
Grams Carb									
Activity									

Date:	Breakfast	Snack	Lunch	Snack	Dinner	Snack	Bedtime	Night	Notes
Blood Sugar									
Insulin Dose									
Grams Carb									
Activity									

Date:	Breakfast	Snack	Lunch	Snack	Dinner	Snack	Bedtime	Night	Notes
Blood Sugar									
Insulin Dose									
Grams Carb									
Activity									

Date:	Breakfast	Snack	Lunch	Snack	Dinner	Snack	Bedtime	Night	Notes
Blood Sugar									
Insulin Dose									
Grams Carb									
Activity									

Weekly Diabetes Record

Name: _____

Date:	Breakfast	Snack	Lunch	Snack	Dinner	Snack	Bedtime	Night	Notes
Blood Sugar									
Insulin Dose									
Grams Carb									
Activity									

Date:	Breakfast	Snack	Lunch	Snack	Dinner	Snack	Bedtime	Night	Notes
Blood Sugar									
Insulin Dose									
Grams Carb									
Activity									

Date:	Breakfast	Snack	Lunch	Snack	Dinner	Snack	Bedtime	Night	Notes
Blood Sugar									
Insulin Dose									
Grams Carb									
Activity									

Date:	Breakfast	Snack	Lunch	Snack	Dinner	Snack	Bedtime	Night	Notes
Blood Sugar									
Insulin Dose									
Grams Carb									
Activity									

Date:	Breakfast	Snack	Lunch	Snack	Dinner	Snack	Bedtime	Night	Notes
Blood Sugar									
Insulin Dose									
Grams Carb									
Activity									

Date:	Breakfast	Snack	Lunch	Snack	Dinner	Snack	Bedtime	Night	Notes
Blood Sugar									
Insulin Dose									
Grams Carb									
Activity									

Date:	Breakfast	Snack	Lunch	Snack	Dinner	Snack	Bedtime	Night	Notes
Blood Sugar									
Insulin Dose									
Grams Carb									
Activity									

Weekly Diabetes Record

Name: _____

Date:	Breakfast	Snack	Lunch	Snack	Dinner	Snack	Bedtime	Night	Notes
Blood Sugar									
Insulin Dose									
Grams Carb									
Activity									

Date:	Breakfast	Snack	Lunch	Snack	Dinner	Snack	Bedtime	Night	Notes
Blood Sugar									
Insulin Dose									
Grams Carb									
Activity									

Date:	Breakfast	Snack	Lunch	Snack	Dinner	Snack	Bedtime	Night	Notes
Blood Sugar									
Insulin Dose									
Grams Carb									
Activity									

Date:	Breakfast	Snack	Lunch	Snack	Dinner	Snack	Bedtime	Night	Notes
Blood Sugar									
Insulin Dose									
Grams Carb									
Activity									

Date:	Breakfast	Snack	Lunch	Snack	Dinner	Snack	Bedtime	Night	Notes
Blood Sugar									
Insulin Dose									
Grams Carb									
Activity									

Date:	Breakfast	Snack	Lunch	Snack	Dinner	Snack	Bedtime	Night	Notes
Blood Sugar									
Insulin Dose									
Grams Carb									
Activity									

Date:	Breakfast	Snack	Lunch	Snack	Dinner	Snack	Bedtime	Night	Notes
Blood Sugar									
Insulin Dose									
Grams Carb									
Activity									

Weekly Diabetes Record

Name: _____

Date:	Breakfast	Snack	Lunch	Snack	Dinner	Snack	Bedtime	Night	Notes
Blood Sugar									
Insulin Dose									
Grams Carb									
Activity									

Date:	Breakfast	Snack	Lunch	Snack	Dinner	Snack	Bedtime	Night	Notes
Blood Sugar									
Insulin Dose									
Grams Carb									
Activity									

Date:	Breakfast	Snack	Lunch	Snack	Dinner	Snack	Bedtime	Night	Notes
Blood Sugar									
Insulin Dose									
Grams Carb									
Activity									

Date:	Breakfast	Snack	Lunch	Snack	Dinner	Snack	Bedtime	Night	Notes
Blood Sugar									
Insulin Dose									
Grams Carb									
Activity									

Date:	Breakfast	Snack	Lunch	Snack	Dinner	Snack	Bedtime	Night	Notes
Blood Sugar									
Insulin Dose									
Grams Carb									
Activity									

Date:	Breakfast	Snack	Lunch	Snack	Dinner	Snack	Bedtime	Night	Notes
Blood Sugar									
Insulin Dose									
Grams Carb									
Activity									

Date:	Breakfast	Snack	Lunch	Snack	Dinner	Snack	Bedtime	Night	Notes
Blood Sugar									
Insulin Dose									
Grams Carb									
Activity									

Weekly Diabetes Record

Name: _____

Date:	Breakfast	Snack	Lunch	Snack	Dinner	Snack	Bedtime	Night	Notes
Blood Sugar									
Insulin Dose									
Grams Carb									
Activity									

Date:	Breakfast	Snack	Lunch	Snack	Dinner	Snack	Bedtime	Night	Notes
Blood Sugar									
Insulin Dose									
Grams Carb									
Activity									

Date:	Breakfast	Snack	Lunch	Snack	Dinner	Snack	Bedtime	Night	Notes
Blood Sugar									
Insulin Dose									
Grams Carb									
Activity									

Date:	Breakfast	Snack	Lunch	Snack	Dinner	Snack	Bedtime	Night	Notes
Blood Sugar									
Insulin Dose									
Grams Carb									
Activity									

Date:	Breakfast	Snack	Lunch	Snack	Dinner	Snack	Bedtime	Night	Notes
Blood Sugar									
Insulin Dose									
Grams Carb									
Activity									

Date:	Breakfast	Snack	Lunch	Snack	Dinner	Snack	Bedtime	Night	Notes
Blood Sugar									
Insulin Dose									
Grams Carb									
Activity									

Date:	Breakfast	Snack	Lunch	Snack	Dinner	Snack	Bedtime	Night	Notes
Blood Sugar									
Insulin Dose									
Grams Carb									
Activity									

Weekly Diabetes Record

Name: _____

Date:	Breakfast	Snack	Lunch	Snack	Dinner	Snack	Bedtime	Night	Notes
Blood Sugar									
Insulin Dose									
Grams Carb									
Activity									

Date:	Breakfast	Snack	Lunch	Snack	Dinner	Snack	Bedtime	Night	Notes
Blood Sugar									
Insulin Dose									
Grams Carb									
Activity									

Date:	Breakfast	Snack	Lunch	Snack	Dinner	Snack	Bedtime	Night	Notes
Blood Sugar									
Insulin Dose									
Grams Carb									
Activity									

Date:	Breakfast	Snack	Lunch	Snack	Dinner	Snack	Bedtime	Night	Notes
Blood Sugar									
Insulin Dose									
Grams Carb									
Activity									

Date:	Breakfast	Snack	Lunch	Snack	Dinner	Snack	Bedtime	Night	Notes
Blood Sugar									
Insulin Dose									
Grams Carb									
Activity									

Date:	Breakfast	Snack	Lunch	Snack	Dinner	Snack	Bedtime	Night	Notes
Blood Sugar									
Insulin Dose									
Grams Carb									
Activity									

Date:	Breakfast	Snack	Lunch	Snack	Dinner	Snack	Bedtime	Night	Notes
Blood Sugar									
Insulin Dose									
Grams Carb									
Activity									

Weekly Diabetes Record

Name: _____

Date:	Breakfast	Snack	Lunch	Snack	Dinner	Snack	Bedtime	Night	Notes
Blood Sugar									
Insulin Dose									
Grams Carb									
Activity									

Date:	Breakfast	Snack	Lunch	Snack	Dinner	Snack	Bedtime	Night	Notes
Blood Sugar									
Insulin Dose									
Grams Carb									
Activity									

Date:	Breakfast	Snack	Lunch	Snack	Dinner	Snack	Bedtime	Night	Notes
Blood Sugar									
Insulin Dose									
Grams Carb									
Activity									

Date:	Breakfast	Snack	Lunch	Snack	Dinner	Snack	Bedtime	Night	Notes
Blood Sugar									
Insulin Dose									
Grams Carb									
Activity									

Date:	Breakfast	Snack	Lunch	Snack	Dinner	Snack	Bedtime	Night	Notes
Blood Sugar									
Insulin Dose									
Grams Carb									
Activity									

Date:	Breakfast	Snack	Lunch	Snack	Dinner	Snack	Bedtime	Night	Notes
Blood Sugar									
Insulin Dose									
Grams Carb									
Activity									

Date:	Breakfast	Snack	Lunch	Snack	Dinner	Snack	Bedtime	Night	Notes
Blood Sugar									
Insulin Dose									
Grams Carb									
Activity									

Weekly Diabetes Record

Name: _____

Date:	Breakfast	Snack	Lunch	Snack	Dinner	Snack	Bedtime	Night	Notes
Blood Sugar									
Insulin Dose									
Grams Carb									
Activity									

Date:	Breakfast	Snack	Lunch	Snack	Dinner	Snack	Bedtime	Night	Notes
Blood Sugar									
Insulin Dose									
Grams Carb									
Activity									

Date:	Breakfast	Snack	Lunch	Snack	Dinner	Snack	Bedtime	Night	Notes
Blood Sugar									
Insulin Dose									
Grams Carb									
Activity									

Date:	Breakfast	Snack	Lunch	Snack	Dinner	Snack	Bedtime	Night	Notes
Blood Sugar									
Insulin Dose									
Grams Carb									
Activity									

Date:	Breakfast	Snack	Lunch	Snack	Dinner	Snack	Bedtime	Night	Notes
Blood Sugar									
Insulin Dose									
Grams Carb									
Activity									

Date:	Breakfast	Snack	Lunch	Snack	Dinner	Snack	Bedtime	Night	Notes
Blood Sugar									
Insulin Dose									
Grams Carb									
Activity									

Date:	Breakfast	Snack	Lunch	Snack	Dinner	Snack	Bedtime	Night	Notes
Blood Sugar									
Insulin Dose									
Grams Carb									
Activity									

Weekly Diabetes Record

Name: _____

Date:	Breakfast	Snack	Lunch	Snack	Dinner	Snack	Bedtime	Night	Notes
Blood Sugar									
Insulin Dose									
Grams Carb									
Activity									

Date:	Breakfast	Snack	Lunch	Snack	Dinner	Snack	Bedtime	Night	Notes
Blood Sugar									
Insulin Dose									
Grams Carb									
Activity									

Date:	Breakfast	Snack	Lunch	Snack	Dinner	Snack	Bedtime	Night	Notes
Blood Sugar									
Insulin Dose									
Grams Carb									
Activity									

Date:	Breakfast	Snack	Lunch	Snack	Dinner	Snack	Bedtime	Night	Notes
Blood Sugar									
Insulin Dose									
Grams Carb									
Activity									

Date:	Breakfast	Snack	Lunch	Snack	Dinner	Snack	Bedtime	Night	Notes
Blood Sugar									
Insulin Dose									
Grams Carb									
Activity									

Date:	Breakfast	Snack	Lunch	Snack	Dinner	Snack	Bedtime	Night	Notes
Blood Sugar									
Insulin Dose									
Grams Carb									
Activity									

Date:	Breakfast	Snack	Lunch	Snack	Dinner	Snack	Bedtime	Night	Notes
Blood Sugar									
Insulin Dose									
Grams Carb									
Activity									

Weekly Diabetes Record

Name: _____

Date:	Breakfast	Snack	Lunch	Snack	Dinner	Snack	Bedtime	Night	Notes
Blood Sugar									
Insulin Dose									
Grams Carb									
Activity									

Date:	Breakfast	Snack	Lunch	Snack	Dinner	Snack	Bedtime	Night	Notes
Blood Sugar									
Insulin Dose									
Grams Carb									
Activity									

Date:	Breakfast	Snack	Lunch	Snack	Dinner	Snack	Bedtime	Night	Notes
Blood Sugar									
Insulin Dose									
Grams Carb									
Activity									

Date:	Breakfast	Snack	Lunch	Snack	Dinner	Snack	Bedtime	Night	Notes
Blood Sugar									
Insulin Dose									
Grams Carb									
Activity									

Date:	Breakfast	Snack	Lunch	Snack	Dinner	Snack	Bedtime	Night	Notes
Blood Sugar									
Insulin Dose									
Grams Carb									
Activity									

Date:	Breakfast	Snack	Lunch	Snack	Dinner	Snack	Bedtime	Night	Notes
Blood Sugar									
Insulin Dose									
Grams Carb									
Activity									

Date:	Breakfast	Snack	Lunch	Snack	Dinner	Snack	Bedtime	Night	Notes
Blood Sugar									
Insulin Dose									
Grams Carb									
Activity									

Weekly Diabetes Record

Name: _____

Date:	Breakfast	Snack	Lunch	Snack	Dinner	Snack	Bedtime	Night	Notes
Blood Sugar									
Insulin Dose									
Grams Carb									
Activity									

Date:	Breakfast	Snack	Lunch	Snack	Dinner	Snack	Bedtime	Night	Notes
Blood Sugar									
Insulin Dose									
Grams Carb									
Activity									

Date:	Breakfast	Snack	Lunch	Snack	Dinner	Snack	Bedtime	Night	Notes
Blood Sugar									
Insulin Dose									
Grams Carb									
Activity									

Date:	Breakfast	Snack	Lunch	Snack	Dinner	Snack	Bedtime	Night	Notes
Blood Sugar									
Insulin Dose									
Grams Carb									
Activity									

Date:	Breakfast	Snack	Lunch	Snack	Dinner	Snack	Bedtime	Night	Notes
Blood Sugar									
Insulin Dose									
Grams Carb									
Activity									

Date:	Breakfast	Snack	Lunch	Snack	Dinner	Snack	Bedtime	Night	Notes
Blood Sugar									
Insulin Dose									
Grams Carb									
Activity									

Date:	Breakfast	Snack	Lunch	Snack	Dinner	Snack	Bedtime	Night	Notes
Blood Sugar									
Insulin Dose									
Grams Carb									
Activity									

Weekly Diabetes Record

Name: _____

Date:	Breakfast	Snack	Lunch	Snack	Dinner	Snack	Bedtime	Night	Notes
Blood Sugar									
Insulin Dose									
Grams Carb									
Activity									

Date:	Breakfast	Snack	Lunch	Snack	Dinner	Snack	Bedtime	Night	Notes
Blood Sugar									
Insulin Dose									
Grams Carb									
Activity									

Date:	Breakfast	Snack	Lunch	Snack	Dinner	Snack	Bedtime	Night	Notes
Blood Sugar									
Insulin Dose									
Grams Carb									
Activity									

Date:	Breakfast	Snack	Lunch	Snack	Dinner	Snack	Bedtime	Night	Notes
Blood Sugar									
Insulin Dose									
Grams Carb									
Activity									

Date:	Breakfast	Snack	Lunch	Snack	Dinner	Snack	Bedtime	Night	Notes
Blood Sugar									
Insulin Dose									
Grams Carb									
Activity									

Date:	Breakfast	Snack	Lunch	Snack	Dinner	Snack	Bedtime	Night	Notes
Blood Sugar									
Insulin Dose									
Grams Carb									
Activity									

Date:	Breakfast	Snack	Lunch	Snack	Dinner	Snack	Bedtime	Night	Notes
Blood Sugar									
Insulin Dose									
Grams Carb									
Activity									

Weekly Diabetes Record

Name: _____

Date:	Breakfast	Snack	Lunch	Snack	Dinner	Snack	Bedtime	Night	Notes
Blood Sugar									
Insulin Dose									
Grams Carb									
Activity									

Date:	Breakfast	Snack	Lunch	Snack	Dinner	Snack	Bedtime	Night	Notes
Blood Sugar									
Insulin Dose									
Grams Carb									
Activity									

Date:	Breakfast	Snack	Lunch	Snack	Dinner	Snack	Bedtime	Night	Notes
Blood Sugar									
Insulin Dose									
Grams Carb									
Activity									

Date:	Breakfast	Snack	Lunch	Snack	Dinner	Snack	Bedtime	Night	Notes
Blood Sugar									
Insulin Dose									
Grams Carb									
Activity									

Date:	Breakfast	Snack	Lunch	Snack	Dinner	Snack	Bedtime	Night	Notes
Blood Sugar									
Insulin Dose									
Grams Carb									
Activity									

Date:	Breakfast	Snack	Lunch	Snack	Dinner	Snack	Bedtime	Night	Notes
Blood Sugar									
Insulin Dose									
Grams Carb									
Activity									

Date:	Breakfast	Snack	Lunch	Snack	Dinner	Snack	Bedtime	Night	Notes
Blood Sugar									
Insulin Dose									
Grams Carb									
Activity									

Weekly Diabetes Record

Name: _____

Date:	Breakfast	Snack	Lunch	Snack	Dinner	Snack	Bedtime	Night	Notes
Blood Sugar									
Insulin Dose									
Grams Carb									
Activity									

Date:	Breakfast	Snack	Lunch	Snack	Dinner	Snack	Bedtime	Night	Notes
Blood Sugar									
Insulin Dose									
Grams Carb									
Activity									

Date:	Breakfast	Snack	Lunch	Snack	Dinner	Snack	Bedtime	Night	Notes
Blood Sugar									
Insulin Dose									
Grams Carb									
Activity									

Date:	Breakfast	Snack	Lunch	Snack	Dinner	Snack	Bedtime	Night	Notes
Blood Sugar									
Insulin Dose									
Grams Carb									
Activity									

Date:	Breakfast	Snack	Lunch	Snack	Dinner	Snack	Bedtime	Night	Notes
Blood Sugar									
Insulin Dose									
Grams Carb									
Activity									

Date:	Breakfast	Snack	Lunch	Snack	Dinner	Snack	Bedtime	Night	Notes
Blood Sugar									
Insulin Dose									
Grams Carb									
Activity									

Date:	Breakfast	Snack	Lunch	Snack	Dinner	Snack	Bedtime	Night	Notes
Blood Sugar									
Insulin Dose									
Grams Carb									
Activity									

Weekly Diabetes Record

Name: _____

Date:	Breakfast	Snack	Lunch	Snack	Dinner	Snack	Bedtime	Night	Notes
Blood Sugar									
Insulin Dose									
Grams Carb									
Activity									

Date:	Breakfast	Snack	Lunch	Snack	Dinner	Snack	Bedtime	Night	Notes
Blood Sugar									
Insulin Dose									
Grams Carb									
Activity									

Date:	Breakfast	Snack	Lunch	Snack	Dinner	Snack	Bedtime	Night	Notes
Blood Sugar									
Insulin Dose									
Grams Carb									
Activity									

Date:	Breakfast	Snack	Lunch	Snack	Dinner	Snack	Bedtime	Night	Notes
Blood Sugar									
Insulin Dose									
Grams Carb									
Activity									

Date:	Breakfast	Snack	Lunch	Snack	Dinner	Snack	Bedtime	Night	Notes
Blood Sugar									
Insulin Dose									
Grams Carb									
Activity									

Date:	Breakfast	Snack	Lunch	Snack	Dinner	Snack	Bedtime	Night	Notes
Blood Sugar									
Insulin Dose									
Grams Carb									
Activity									

Date:	Breakfast	Snack	Lunch	Snack	Dinner	Snack	Bedtime	Night	Notes
Blood Sugar									
Insulin Dose									
Grams Carb									
Activity									

Weekly Diabetes Record

Name: _____

Date:	Breakfast	Snack	Lunch	Snack	Dinner	Snack	Bedtime	Night	Notes
Blood Sugar									
Insulin Dose									
Grams Carb									
Activity									

Date:	Breakfast	Snack	Lunch	Snack	Dinner	Snack	Bedtime	Night	Notes
Blood Sugar									
Insulin Dose									
Grams Carb									
Activity									

Date:	Breakfast	Snack	Lunch	Snack	Dinner	Snack	Bedtime	Night	Notes
Blood Sugar									
Insulin Dose									
Grams Carb									
Activity									

Date:	Breakfast	Snack	Lunch	Snack	Dinner	Snack	Bedtime	Night	Notes
Blood Sugar									
Insulin Dose									
Grams Carb									
Activity									

Date:	Breakfast	Snack	Lunch	Snack	Dinner	Snack	Bedtime	Night	Notes
Blood Sugar									
Insulin Dose									
Grams Carb									
Activity									

Date:	Breakfast	Snack	Lunch	Snack	Dinner	Snack	Bedtime	Night	Notes
Blood Sugar									
Insulin Dose									
Grams Carb									
Activity									

Date:	Breakfast	Snack	Lunch	Snack	Dinner	Snack	Bedtime	Night	Notes
Blood Sugar									
Insulin Dose									
Grams Carb									
Activity									

Weekly Diabetes Record

Name: _____

Date:	Breakfast	Snack	Lunch	Snack	Dinner	Snack	Bedtime	Night	Notes
Blood Sugar									
Insulin Dose									
Grams Carb									
Activity									

Date:	Breakfast	Snack	Lunch	Snack	Dinner	Snack	Bedtime	Night	Notes
Blood Sugar									
Insulin Dose									
Grams Carb									
Activity									

Date:	Breakfast	Snack	Lunch	Snack	Dinner	Snack	Bedtime	Night	Notes
Blood Sugar									
Insulin Dose									
Grams Carb									
Activity									

Date:	Breakfast	Snack	Lunch	Snack	Dinner	Snack	Bedtime	Night	Notes
Blood Sugar									
Insulin Dose									
Grams Carb									
Activity									

Date:	Breakfast	Snack	Lunch	Snack	Dinner	Snack	Bedtime	Night	Notes
Blood Sugar									
Insulin Dose									
Grams Carb									
Activity									

Date:	Breakfast	Snack	Lunch	Snack	Dinner	Snack	Bedtime	Night	Notes
Blood Sugar									
Insulin Dose									
Grams Carb									
Activity									

Date:	Breakfast	Snack	Lunch	Snack	Dinner	Snack	Bedtime	Night	Notes
Blood Sugar									
Insulin Dose									
Grams Carb									
Activity									

Weekly Diabetes Record

Name: _____

Date:	Breakfast	Snack	Lunch	Snack	Dinner	Snack	Bedtime	Night	Notes
Blood Sugar									
Insulin Dose									
Grams Carb									
Activity									

Date:	Breakfast	Snack	Lunch	Snack	Dinner	Snack	Bedtime	Night	Notes
Blood Sugar									
Insulin Dose									
Grams Carb									
Activity									

Date:	Breakfast	Snack	Lunch	Snack	Dinner	Snack	Bedtime	Night	Notes
Blood Sugar									
Insulin Dose									
Grams Carb									
Activity									

Date:	Breakfast	Snack	Lunch	Snack	Dinner	Snack	Bedtime	Night	Notes
Blood Sugar									
Insulin Dose									
Grams Carb									
Activity									

Date:	Breakfast	Snack	Lunch	Snack	Dinner	Snack	Bedtime	Night	Notes
Blood Sugar									
Insulin Dose									
Grams Carb									
Activity									

Date:	Breakfast	Snack	Lunch	Snack	Dinner	Snack	Bedtime	Night	Notes
Blood Sugar									
Insulin Dose									
Grams Carb									
Activity									

Date:	Breakfast	Snack	Lunch	Snack	Dinner	Snack	Bedtime	Night	Notes
Blood Sugar									
Insulin Dose									
Grams Carb									
Activity									

Weekly Diabetes Record

Name: _____

Date:	Breakfast	Snack	Lunch	Snack	Dinner	Snack	Bedtime	Night	Notes
Blood Sugar									
Insulin Dose									
Grams Carb									
Activity									

Date:	Breakfast	Snack	Lunch	Snack	Dinner	Snack	Bedtime	Night	Notes
Blood Sugar									
Insulin Dose									
Grams Carb									
Activity									

Date:	Breakfast	Snack	Lunch	Snack	Dinner	Snack	Bedtime	Night	Notes
Blood Sugar									
Insulin Dose									
Grams Carb									
Activity									

Date:	Breakfast	Snack	Lunch	Snack	Dinner	Snack	Bedtime	Night	Notes
Blood Sugar									
Insulin Dose									
Grams Carb									
Activity									

Date:	Breakfast	Snack	Lunch	Snack	Dinner	Snack	Bedtime	Night	Notes
Blood Sugar									
Insulin Dose									
Grams Carb									
Activity									

Date:	Breakfast	Snack	Lunch	Snack	Dinner	Snack	Bedtime	Night	Notes
Blood Sugar									
Insulin Dose									
Grams Carb									
Activity									

Date:	Breakfast	Snack	Lunch	Snack	Dinner	Snack	Bedtime	Night	Notes
Blood Sugar									
Insulin Dose									
Grams Carb									
Activity									

Weekly Diabetes Record

Name: _____

Date:	Breakfast	Snack	Lunch	Snack	Dinner	Snack	Bedtime	Night	Notes
Blood Sugar									
Insulin Dose									
Grams Carb									
Activity									

Date:	Breakfast	Snack	Lunch	Snack	Dinner	Snack	Bedtime	Night	Notes
Blood Sugar									
Insulin Dose									
Grams Carb									
Activity									

Date:	Breakfast	Snack	Lunch	Snack	Dinner	Snack	Bedtime	Night	Notes
Blood Sugar									
Insulin Dose									
Grams Carb									
Activity									

Date:	Breakfast	Snack	Lunch	Snack	Dinner	Snack	Bedtime	Night	Notes
Blood Sugar									
Insulin Dose									
Grams Carb									
Activity									

Date:	Breakfast	Snack	Lunch	Snack	Dinner	Snack	Bedtime	Night	Notes
Blood Sugar									
Insulin Dose									
Grams Carb									
Activity									

Date:	Breakfast	Snack	Lunch	Snack	Dinner	Snack	Bedtime	Night	Notes
Blood Sugar									
Insulin Dose									
Grams Carb									
Activity									

Date:	Breakfast	Snack	Lunch	Snack	Dinner	Snack	Bedtime	Night	Notes
Blood Sugar									
Insulin Dose									
Grams Carb									
Activity									

Weekly Diabetes Record

Name: _____

Date:	Breakfast	Snack	Lunch	Snack	Dinner	Snack	Bedtime	Night	Notes
Blood Sugar									
Insulin Dose									
Grams Carb									
Activity									

Date:	Breakfast	Snack	Lunch	Snack	Dinner	Snack	Bedtime	Night	Notes
Blood Sugar									
Insulin Dose									
Grams Carb									
Activity									

Date:	Breakfast	Snack	Lunch	Snack	Dinner	Snack	Bedtime	Night	Notes
Blood Sugar									
Insulin Dose									
Grams Carb									
Activity									

Date:	Breakfast	Snack	Lunch	Snack	Dinner	Snack	Bedtime	Night	Notes
Blood Sugar									
Insulin Dose									
Grams Carb									
Activity									

Date:	Breakfast	Snack	Lunch	Snack	Dinner	Snack	Bedtime	Night	Notes
Blood Sugar									
Insulin Dose									
Grams Carb									
Activity									

Date:	Breakfast	Snack	Lunch	Snack	Dinner	Snack	Bedtime	Night	Notes
Blood Sugar									
Insulin Dose									
Grams Carb									
Activity									

Date:	Breakfast	Snack	Lunch	Snack	Dinner	Snack	Bedtime	Night	Notes
Blood Sugar									
Insulin Dose									
Grams Carb									
Activity									

Weekly Diabetes Record

Name: _____

Date:	Breakfast	Snack	Lunch	Snack	Dinner	Snack	Bedtime	Night	Notes
Blood Sugar									
Insulin Dose									
Grams Carb									
Activity									

Date:	Breakfast	Snack	Lunch	Snack	Dinner	Snack	Bedtime	Night	Notes
Blood Sugar									
Insulin Dose									
Grams Carb									
Activity									

Date:	Breakfast	Snack	Lunch	Snack	Dinner	Snack	Bedtime	Night	Notes
Blood Sugar									
Insulin Dose									
Grams Carb									
Activity									

Date:	Breakfast	Snack	Lunch	Snack	Dinner	Snack	Bedtime	Night	Notes
Blood Sugar									
Insulin Dose									
Grams Carb									
Activity									

Date:	Breakfast	Snack	Lunch	Snack	Dinner	Snack	Bedtime	Night	Notes
Blood Sugar									
Insulin Dose									
Grams Carb									
Activity									

Date:	Breakfast	Snack	Lunch	Snack	Dinner	Snack	Bedtime	Night	Notes
Blood Sugar									
Insulin Dose									
Grams Carb									
Activity									

Date:	Breakfast	Snack	Lunch	Snack	Dinner	Snack	Bedtime	Night	Notes
Blood Sugar									
Insulin Dose									
Grams Carb									
Activity									

Weekly Diabetes Record

Name: _____

Date:	Breakfast	Snack	Lunch	Snack	Dinner	Snack	Bedtime	Night	Notes
Blood Sugar									
Insulin Dose									
Grams Carb									
Activity									

Date:	Breakfast	Snack	Lunch	Snack	Dinner	Snack	Bedtime	Night	Notes
Blood Sugar									
Insulin Dose									
Grams Carb									
Activity									

Date:	Breakfast	Snack	Lunch	Snack	Dinner	Snack	Bedtime	Night	Notes
Blood Sugar									
Insulin Dose									
Grams Carb									
Activity									

Date:	Breakfast	Snack	Lunch	Snack	Dinner	Snack	Bedtime	Night	Notes
Blood Sugar									
Insulin Dose									
Grams Carb									
Activity									

Date:	Breakfast	Snack	Lunch	Snack	Dinner	Snack	Bedtime	Night	Notes
Blood Sugar									
Insulin Dose									
Grams Carb									
Activity									

Date:	Breakfast	Snack	Lunch	Snack	Dinner	Snack	Bedtime	Night	Notes
Blood Sugar									
Insulin Dose									
Grams Carb									
Activity									

Date:	Breakfast	Snack	Lunch	Snack	Dinner	Snack	Bedtime	Night	Notes
Blood Sugar									
Insulin Dose									
Grams Carb									
Activity									

Weekly Diabetes Record

Name: _____

Date:	Breakfast	Snack	Lunch	Snack	Dinner	Snack	Bedtime	Night	Notes
Blood Sugar									
Insulin Dose									
Grams Carb									
Activity									

Date:	Breakfast	Snack	Lunch	Snack	Dinner	Snack	Bedtime	Night	Notes
Blood Sugar									
Insulin Dose									
Grams Carb									
Activity									

Date:	Breakfast	Snack	Lunch	Snack	Dinner	Snack	Bedtime	Night	Notes
Blood Sugar									
Insulin Dose									
Grams Carb									
Activity									

Date:	Breakfast	Snack	Lunch	Snack	Dinner	Snack	Bedtime	Night	Notes
Blood Sugar									
Insulin Dose									
Grams Carb									
Activity									

Date:	Breakfast	Snack	Lunch	Snack	Dinner	Snack	Bedtime	Night	Notes
Blood Sugar									
Insulin Dose									
Grams Carb									
Activity									

Date:	Breakfast	Snack	Lunch	Snack	Dinner	Snack	Bedtime	Night	Notes
Blood Sugar									
Insulin Dose									
Grams Carb									
Activity									

Date:	Breakfast	Snack	Lunch	Snack	Dinner	Snack	Bedtime	Night	Notes
Blood Sugar									
Insulin Dose									
Grams Carb									
Activity									

Weekly Diabetes Record

Name: _____

Date:	Breakfast	Snack	Lunch	Snack	Dinner	Snack	Bedtime	Night	Notes
Blood Sugar									
Insulin Dose									
Grams Carb									
Activity									

Date:	Breakfast	Snack	Lunch	Snack	Dinner	Snack	Bedtime	Night	Notes
Blood Sugar									
Insulin Dose									
Grams Carb									
Activity									

Date:	Breakfast	Snack	Lunch	Snack	Dinner	Snack	Bedtime	Night	Notes
Blood Sugar									
Insulin Dose									
Grams Carb									
Activity									

Date:	Breakfast	Snack	Lunch	Snack	Dinner	Snack	Bedtime	Night	Notes
Blood Sugar									
Insulin Dose									
Grams Carb									
Activity									

Date:	Breakfast	Snack	Lunch	Snack	Dinner	Snack	Bedtime	Night	Notes
Blood Sugar									
Insulin Dose									
Grams Carb									
Activity									

Date:	Breakfast	Snack	Lunch	Snack	Dinner	Snack	Bedtime	Night	Notes
Blood Sugar									
Insulin Dose									
Grams Carb									
Activity									

Date:	Breakfast	Snack	Lunch	Snack	Dinner	Snack	Bedtime	Night	Notes
Blood Sugar									
Insulin Dose									
Grams Carb									
Activity									

Weekly Diabetes Record

Name: _____

Date:	Breakfast	Snack	Lunch	Snack	Dinner	Snack	Bedtime	Night	Notes
Blood Sugar									
Insulin Dose									
Grams Carb									
Activity									

Date:	Breakfast	Snack	Lunch	Snack	Dinner	Snack	Bedtime	Night	Notes
Blood Sugar									
Insulin Dose									
Grams Carb									
Activity									

Date:	Breakfast	Snack	Lunch	Snack	Dinner	Snack	Bedtime	Night	Notes
Blood Sugar									
Insulin Dose									
Grams Carb									
Activity									

Date:	Breakfast	Snack	Lunch	Snack	Dinner	Snack	Bedtime	Night	Notes
Blood Sugar									
Insulin Dose									
Grams Carb									
Activity									

Date:	Breakfast	Snack	Lunch	Snack	Dinner	Snack	Bedtime	Night	Notes
Blood Sugar									
Insulin Dose									
Grams Carb									
Activity									

Date:	Breakfast	Snack	Lunch	Snack	Dinner	Snack	Bedtime	Night	Notes
Blood Sugar									
Insulin Dose									
Grams Carb									
Activity									

Date:	Breakfast	Snack	Lunch	Snack	Dinner	Snack	Bedtime	Night	Notes
Blood Sugar									
Insulin Dose									
Grams Carb									
Activity									

Weekly Diabetes Record

Name: _____

Date:	Breakfast	Snack	Lunch	Snack	Dinner	Snack	Bedtime	Night	Notes
Blood Sugar									
Insulin Dose									
Grams Carb									
Activity									

Date:	Breakfast	Snack	Lunch	Snack	Dinner	Snack	Bedtime	Night	Notes
Blood Sugar									
Insulin Dose									
Grams Carb									
Activity									

Date:	Breakfast	Snack	Lunch	Snack	Dinner	Snack	Bedtime	Night	Notes
Blood Sugar									
Insulin Dose									
Grams Carb									
Activity									

Date:	Breakfast	Snack	Lunch	Snack	Dinner	Snack	Bedtime	Night	Notes
Blood Sugar									
Insulin Dose									
Grams Carb									
Activity									

Date:	Breakfast	Snack	Lunch	Snack	Dinner	Snack	Bedtime	Night	Notes
Blood Sugar									
Insulin Dose									
Grams Carb									
Activity									

Date:	Breakfast	Snack	Lunch	Snack	Dinner	Snack	Bedtime	Night	Notes
Blood Sugar									
Insulin Dose									
Grams Carb									
Activity									

Date:	Breakfast	Snack	Lunch	Snack	Dinner	Snack	Bedtime	Night	Notes
Blood Sugar									
Insulin Dose									
Grams Carb									
Activity									

Weekly Diabetes Record

Name: _____

Date:	Breakfast	Snack	Lunch	Snack	Dinner	Snack	Bedtime	Night	Notes
Blood Sugar									
Insulin Dose									
Grams Carb									
Activity									

Date:	Breakfast	Snack	Lunch	Snack	Dinner	Snack	Bedtime	Night	Notes
Blood Sugar									
Insulin Dose									
Grams Carb									
Activity									

Date:	Breakfast	Snack	Lunch	Snack	Dinner	Snack	Bedtime	Night	Notes
Blood Sugar									
Insulin Dose									
Grams Carb									
Activity									

Date:	Breakfast	Snack	Lunch	Snack	Dinner	Snack	Bedtime	Night	Notes
Blood Sugar									
Insulin Dose									
Grams Carb									
Activity									

Date:	Breakfast	Snack	Lunch	Snack	Dinner	Snack	Bedtime	Night	Notes
Blood Sugar									
Insulin Dose									
Grams Carb									
Activity									

Date:	Breakfast	Snack	Lunch	Snack	Dinner	Snack	Bedtime	Night	Notes
Blood Sugar									
Insulin Dose									
Grams Carb									
Activity									

Date:	Breakfast	Snack	Lunch	Snack	Dinner	Snack	Bedtime	Night	Notes
Blood Sugar									
Insulin Dose									
Grams Carb									
Activity									

Weekly Diabetes Record

Name: _____

Date:	Breakfast	Snack	Lunch	Snack	Dinner	Snack	Bedtime	Night	Notes
Blood Sugar									
Insulin Dose									
Grams Carb									
Activity									

Date:	Breakfast	Snack	Lunch	Snack	Dinner	Snack	Bedtime	Night	Notes
Blood Sugar									
Insulin Dose									
Grams Carb									
Activity									

Date:	Breakfast	Snack	Lunch	Snack	Dinner	Snack	Bedtime	Night	Notes
Blood Sugar									
Insulin Dose									
Grams Carb									
Activity									

Date:	Breakfast	Snack	Lunch	Snack	Dinner	Snack	Bedtime	Night	Notes
Blood Sugar									
Insulin Dose									
Grams Carb									
Activity									

Date:	Breakfast	Snack	Lunch	Snack	Dinner	Snack	Bedtime	Night	Notes
Blood Sugar									
Insulin Dose									
Grams Carb									
Activity									

Date:	Breakfast	Snack	Lunch	Snack	Dinner	Snack	Bedtime	Night	Notes
Blood Sugar									
Insulin Dose									
Grams Carb									
Activity									

Date:	Breakfast	Snack	Lunch	Snack	Dinner	Snack	Bedtime	Night	Notes
Blood Sugar									
Insulin Dose									
Grams Carb									
Activity									

Weekly Diabetes Record

Name: _____

Date:	Breakfast	Snack	Lunch	Snack	Dinner	Snack	Bedtime	Night	Notes
Blood Sugar									
Insulin Dose									
Grams Carb									
Activity									

Date:	Breakfast	Snack	Lunch	Snack	Dinner	Snack	Bedtime	Night	Notes
Blood Sugar									
Insulin Dose									
Grams Carb									
Activity									

Date:	Breakfast	Snack	Lunch	Snack	Dinner	Snack	Bedtime	Night	Notes
Blood Sugar									
Insulin Dose									
Grams Carb									
Activity									

Date:	Breakfast	Snack	Lunch	Snack	Dinner	Snack	Bedtime	Night	Notes
Blood Sugar									
Insulin Dose									
Grams Carb									
Activity									

Date:	Breakfast	Snack	Lunch	Snack	Dinner	Snack	Bedtime	Night	Notes
Blood Sugar									
Insulin Dose									
Grams Carb									
Activity									

Date:	Breakfast	Snack	Lunch	Snack	Dinner	Snack	Bedtime	Night	Notes
Blood Sugar									
Insulin Dose									
Grams Carb									
Activity									

Date:	Breakfast	Snack	Lunch	Snack	Dinner	Snack	Bedtime	Night	Notes
Blood Sugar									
Insulin Dose									
Grams Carb									
Activity									

Weekly Diabetes Record

Name: _____

Date:	Breakfast	Snack	Lunch	Snack	Dinner	Snack	Bedtime	Night	Notes
Blood Sugar									
Insulin Dose									
Grams Carb									
Activity									

Date:	Breakfast	Snack	Lunch	Snack	Dinner	Snack	Bedtime	Night	Notes
Blood Sugar									
Insulin Dose									
Grams Carb									
Activity									

Date:	Breakfast	Snack	Lunch	Snack	Dinner	Snack	Bedtime	Night	Notes
Blood Sugar									
Insulin Dose									
Grams Carb									
Activity									

Date:	Breakfast	Snack	Lunch	Snack	Dinner	Snack	Bedtime	Night	Notes
Blood Sugar									
Insulin Dose									
Grams Carb									
Activity									

Date:	Breakfast	Snack	Lunch	Snack	Dinner	Snack	Bedtime	Night	Notes
Blood Sugar									
Insulin Dose									
Grams Carb									
Activity									

Date:	Breakfast	Snack	Lunch	Snack	Dinner	Snack	Bedtime	Night	Notes
Blood Sugar									
Insulin Dose									
Grams Carb									
Activity									

Date:	Breakfast	Snack	Lunch	Snack	Dinner	Snack	Bedtime	Night	Notes
Blood Sugar									
Insulin Dose									
Grams Carb									
Activity									

Weekly Diabetes Record

Name: _____

Date:	Breakfast	Snack	Lunch	Snack	Dinner	Snack	Bedtime	Night	Notes
Blood Sugar									
Insulin Dose									
Grams Carb									
Activity									

Date:	Breakfast	Snack	Lunch	Snack	Dinner	Snack	Bedtime	Night	Notes
Blood Sugar									
Insulin Dose									
Grams Carb									
Activity									

Date:	Breakfast	Snack	Lunch	Snack	Dinner	Snack	Bedtime	Night	Notes
Blood Sugar									
Insulin Dose									
Grams Carb									
Activity									

Date:	Breakfast	Snack	Lunch	Snack	Dinner	Snack	Bedtime	Night	Notes
Blood Sugar									
Insulin Dose									
Grams Carb									
Activity									

Date:	Breakfast	Snack	Lunch	Snack	Dinner	Snack	Bedtime	Night	Notes
Blood Sugar									
Insulin Dose									
Grams Carb									
Activity									

Date:	Breakfast	Snack	Lunch	Snack	Dinner	Snack	Bedtime	Night	Notes
Blood Sugar									
Insulin Dose									
Grams Carb									
Activity									

Date:	Breakfast	Snack	Lunch	Snack	Dinner	Snack	Bedtime	Night	Notes
Blood Sugar									
Insulin Dose									
Grams Carb									
Activity									

Weekly Diabetes Record

Name: _____

Date:	Breakfast	Snack	Lunch	Snack	Dinner	Snack	Bedtime	Night	Notes
Blood Sugar									
Insulin Dose									
Grams Carb									
Activity									

Date:	Breakfast	Snack	Lunch	Snack	Dinner	Snack	Bedtime	Night	Notes
Blood Sugar									
Insulin Dose									
Grams Carb									
Activity									

Date:	Breakfast	Snack	Lunch	Snack	Dinner	Snack	Bedtime	Night	Notes
Blood Sugar									
Insulin Dose									
Grams Carb									
Activity									

Date:	Breakfast	Snack	Lunch	Snack	Dinner	Snack	Bedtime	Night	Notes
Blood Sugar									
Insulin Dose									
Grams Carb									
Activity									

Date:	Breakfast	Snack	Lunch	Snack	Dinner	Snack	Bedtime	Night	Notes
Blood Sugar									
Insulin Dose									
Grams Carb									
Activity									

Date:	Breakfast	Snack	Lunch	Snack	Dinner	Snack	Bedtime	Night	Notes
Blood Sugar									
Insulin Dose									
Grams Carb									
Activity									

Date:	Breakfast	Snack	Lunch	Snack	Dinner	Snack	Bedtime	Night	Notes
Blood Sugar									
Insulin Dose									
Grams Carb									
Activity									

Weekly Diabetes Record

Name: _____

Date:	Breakfast	Snack	Lunch	Snack	Dinner	Snack	Bedtime	Night	Notes
Blood Sugar									
Insulin Dose									
Grams Carb									
Activity									

Date:	Breakfast	Snack	Lunch	Snack	Dinner	Snack	Bedtime	Night	Notes
Blood Sugar									
Insulin Dose									
Grams Carb									
Activity									

Date:	Breakfast	Snack	Lunch	Snack	Dinner	Snack	Bedtime	Night	Notes
Blood Sugar									
Insulin Dose									
Grams Carb									
Activity									

Date:	Breakfast	Snack	Lunch	Snack	Dinner	Snack	Bedtime	Night	Notes
Blood Sugar									
Insulin Dose									
Grams Carb									
Activity									

Date:	Breakfast	Snack	Lunch	Snack	Dinner	Snack	Bedtime	Night	Notes
Blood Sugar									
Insulin Dose									
Grams Carb									
Activity									

Date:	Breakfast	Snack	Lunch	Snack	Dinner	Snack	Bedtime	Night	Notes
Blood Sugar									
Insulin Dose									
Grams Carb									
Activity									

Date:	Breakfast	Snack	Lunch	Snack	Dinner	Snack	Bedtime	Night	Notes
Blood Sugar									
Insulin Dose									
Grams Carb									
Activity									

Weekly Diabetes Record

Name: _____

Date:	Breakfast	Snack	Lunch	Snack	Dinner	Snack	Bedtime	Night	Notes
Blood Sugar									
Insulin Dose									
Grams Carb									
Activity									

Date:	Breakfast	Snack	Lunch	Snack	Dinner	Snack	Bedtime	Night	Notes
Blood Sugar									
Insulin Dose									
Grams Carb									
Activity									

Date:	Breakfast	Snack	Lunch	Snack	Dinner	Snack	Bedtime	Night	Notes
Blood Sugar									
Insulin Dose									
Grams Carb									
Activity									

Date:	Breakfast	Snack	Lunch	Snack	Dinner	Snack	Bedtime	Night	Notes
Blood Sugar									
Insulin Dose									
Grams Carb									
Activity									

Date:	Breakfast	Snack	Lunch	Snack	Dinner	Snack	Bedtime	Night	Notes
Blood Sugar									
Insulin Dose									
Grams Carb									
Activity									

Date:	Breakfast	Snack	Lunch	Snack	Dinner	Snack	Bedtime	Night	Notes
Blood Sugar									
Insulin Dose									
Grams Carb									
Activity									

Date:	Breakfast	Snack	Lunch	Snack	Dinner	Snack	Bedtime	Night	Notes
Blood Sugar									
Insulin Dose									
Grams Carb									
Activity									

Weekly Diabetes Record

Name: _____

Date:	Breakfast	Snack	Lunch	Snack	Dinner	Snack	Bedtime	Night	Notes
Blood Sugar									
Insulin Dose									
Grams Carb									
Activity									

Date:	Breakfast	Snack	Lunch	Snack	Dinner	Snack	Bedtime	Night	Notes
Blood Sugar									
Insulin Dose									
Grams Carb									
Activity									

Date:	Breakfast	Snack	Lunch	Snack	Dinner	Snack	Bedtime	Night	Notes
Blood Sugar									
Insulin Dose									
Grams Carb									
Activity									

Date:	Breakfast	Snack	Lunch	Snack	Dinner	Snack	Bedtime	Night	Notes
Blood Sugar									
Insulin Dose									
Grams Carb									
Activity									

Date:	Breakfast	Snack	Lunch	Snack	Dinner	Snack	Bedtime	Night	Notes
Blood Sugar									
Insulin Dose									
Grams Carb									
Activity									

Date:	Breakfast	Snack	Lunch	Snack	Dinner	Snack	Bedtime	Night	Notes
Blood Sugar									
Insulin Dose									
Grams Carb									
Activity									

Date:	Breakfast	Snack	Lunch	Snack	Dinner	Snack	Bedtime	Night	Notes
Blood Sugar									
Insulin Dose									
Grams Carb									
Activity									

Weekly Diabetes Record

Name: _____

Date:	Breakfast	Snack	Lunch	Snack	Dinner	Snack	Bedtime	Night	Notes
Blood Sugar									
Insulin Dose									
Grams Carb									
Activity									

Date:	Breakfast	Snack	Lunch	Snack	Dinner	Snack	Bedtime	Night	Notes
Blood Sugar									
Insulin Dose									
Grams Carb									
Activity									

Date:	Breakfast	Snack	Lunch	Snack	Dinner	Snack	Bedtime	Night	Notes
Blood Sugar									
Insulin Dose									
Grams Carb									
Activity									

Date:	Breakfast	Snack	Lunch	Snack	Dinner	Snack	Bedtime	Night	Notes
Blood Sugar									
Insulin Dose									
Grams Carb									
Activity									

Date:	Breakfast	Snack	Lunch	Snack	Dinner	Snack	Bedtime	Night	Notes
Blood Sugar									
Insulin Dose									
Grams Carb									
Activity									

Date:	Breakfast	Snack	Lunch	Snack	Dinner	Snack	Bedtime	Night	Notes
Blood Sugar									
Insulin Dose									
Grams Carb									
Activity									

Date:	Breakfast	Snack	Lunch	Snack	Dinner	Snack	Bedtime	Night	Notes
Blood Sugar									
Insulin Dose									
Grams Carb									
Activity									

Weekly Diabetes Record

Name: _____

Date:	Breakfast	Snack	Lunch	Snack	Dinner	Snack	Bedtime	Night	Notes
Blood Sugar									
Insulin Dose									
Grams Carb									
Activity									

Date:	Breakfast	Snack	Lunch	Snack	Dinner	Snack	Bedtime	Night	Notes
Blood Sugar									
Insulin Dose									
Grams Carb									
Activity									

Date:	Breakfast	Snack	Lunch	Snack	Dinner	Snack	Bedtime	Night	Notes
Blood Sugar									
Insulin Dose									
Grams Carb									
Activity									

Date:	Breakfast	Snack	Lunch	Snack	Dinner	Snack	Bedtime	Night	Notes
Blood Sugar									
Insulin Dose									
Grams Carb									
Activity									

Date:	Breakfast	Snack	Lunch	Snack	Dinner	Snack	Bedtime	Night	Notes
Blood Sugar									
Insulin Dose									
Grams Carb									
Activity									

Date:	Breakfast	Snack	Lunch	Snack	Dinner	Snack	Bedtime	Night	Notes
Blood Sugar									
Insulin Dose									
Grams Carb									
Activity									

Date:	Breakfast	Snack	Lunch	Snack	Dinner	Snack	Bedtime	Night	Notes
Blood Sugar									
Insulin Dose									
Grams Carb									
Activity									

Weekly Diabetes Record

Name: _____

Date:	Breakfast	Snack	Lunch	Snack	Dinner	Snack	Bedtime	Night	Notes
Blood Sugar									
Insulin Dose									
Grams Carb									
Activity									

Date:	Breakfast	Snack	Lunch	Snack	Dinner	Snack	Bedtime	Night	Notes
Blood Sugar									
Insulin Dose									
Grams Carb									
Activity									

Date:	Breakfast	Snack	Lunch	Snack	Dinner	Snack	Bedtime	Night	Notes
Blood Sugar									
Insulin Dose									
Grams Carb									
Activity									

Date:	Breakfast	Snack	Lunch	Snack	Dinner	Snack	Bedtime	Night	Notes
Blood Sugar									
Insulin Dose									
Grams Carb									
Activity									

Date:	Breakfast	Snack	Lunch	Snack	Dinner	Snack	Bedtime	Night	Notes
Blood Sugar									
Insulin Dose									
Grams Carb									
Activity									

Date:	Breakfast	Snack	Lunch	Snack	Dinner	Snack	Bedtime	Night	Notes
Blood Sugar									
Insulin Dose									
Grams Carb									
Activity									

Date:	Breakfast	Snack	Lunch	Snack	Dinner	Snack	Bedtime	Night	Notes
Blood Sugar									
Insulin Dose									
Grams Carb									
Activity									

Weekly Diabetes Record

Name: _____

Date:	Breakfast	Snack	Lunch	Snack	Dinner	Snack	Bedtime	Night	Notes
Blood Sugar									
Insulin Dose									
Grams Carb									
Activity									

Date:	Breakfast	Snack	Lunch	Snack	Dinner	Snack	Bedtime	Night	Notes
Blood Sugar									
Insulin Dose									
Grams Carb									
Activity									

Date:	Breakfast	Snack	Lunch	Snack	Dinner	Snack	Bedtime	Night	Notes
Blood Sugar									
Insulin Dose									
Grams Carb									
Activity									

Date:	Breakfast	Snack	Lunch	Snack	Dinner	Snack	Bedtime	Night	Notes
Blood Sugar									
Insulin Dose									
Grams Carb									
Activity									

Date:	Breakfast	Snack	Lunch	Snack	Dinner	Snack	Bedtime	Night	Notes
Blood Sugar									
Insulin Dose									
Grams Carb									
Activity									

Date:	Breakfast	Snack	Lunch	Snack	Dinner	Snack	Bedtime	Night	Notes
Blood Sugar									
Insulin Dose									
Grams Carb									
Activity									

Date:	Breakfast	Snack	Lunch	Snack	Dinner	Snack	Bedtime	Night	Notes
Blood Sugar									
Insulin Dose									
Grams Carb									
Activity									

Weekly Diabetes Record

Name: _____

Date:	Breakfast	Snack	Lunch	Snack	Dinner	Snack	Bedtime	Night	Notes
Blood Sugar									
Insulin Dose									
Grams Carb									
Activity									

Date:	Breakfast	Snack	Lunch	Snack	Dinner	Snack	Bedtime	Night	Notes
Blood Sugar									
Insulin Dose									
Grams Carb									
Activity									

Date:	Breakfast	Snack	Lunch	Snack	Dinner	Snack	Bedtime	Night	Notes
Blood Sugar									
Insulin Dose									
Grams Carb									
Activity									

Date:	Breakfast	Snack	Lunch	Snack	Dinner	Snack	Bedtime	Night	Notes
Blood Sugar									
Insulin Dose									
Grams Carb									
Activity									

Date:	Breakfast	Snack	Lunch	Snack	Dinner	Snack	Bedtime	Night	Notes
Blood Sugar									
Insulin Dose									
Grams Carb									
Activity									

Date:	Breakfast	Snack	Lunch	Snack	Dinner	Snack	Bedtime	Night	Notes
Blood Sugar									
Insulin Dose									
Grams Carb									
Activity									

Date:	Breakfast	Snack	Lunch	Snack	Dinner	Snack	Bedtime	Night	Notes
Blood Sugar									
Insulin Dose									
Grams Carb									
Activity									

Weekly Diabetes Record

Name: _____

Date:	Breakfast	Snack	Lunch	Snack	Dinner	Snack	Bedtime	Night	Notes
Blood Sugar									
Insulin Dose									
Grams Carb									
Activity									

Date:	Breakfast	Snack	Lunch	Snack	Dinner	Snack	Bedtime	Night	Notes
Blood Sugar									
Insulin Dose									
Grams Carb									
Activity									

Date:	Breakfast	Snack	Lunch	Snack	Dinner	Snack	Bedtime	Night	Notes
Blood Sugar									
Insulin Dose									
Grams Carb									
Activity									

Date:	Breakfast	Snack	Lunch	Snack	Dinner	Snack	Bedtime	Night	Notes
Blood Sugar									
Insulin Dose									
Grams Carb									
Activity									

Date:	Breakfast	Snack	Lunch	Snack	Dinner	Snack	Bedtime	Night	Notes
Blood Sugar									
Insulin Dose									
Grams Carb									
Activity									

Date:	Breakfast	Snack	Lunch	Snack	Dinner	Snack	Bedtime	Night	Notes
Blood Sugar									
Insulin Dose									
Grams Carb									
Activity									

Date:	Breakfast	Snack	Lunch	Snack	Dinner	Snack	Bedtime	Night	Notes
Blood Sugar									
Insulin Dose									
Grams Carb									
Activity									

Weekly Diabetes Record

Name: _____

Date:	Breakfast	Snack	Lunch	Snack	Dinner	Snack	Bedtime	Night	Notes
Blood Sugar									
Insulin Dose									
Grams Carb									
Activity									

Date:	Breakfast	Snack	Lunch	Snack	Dinner	Snack	Bedtime	Night	Notes
Blood Sugar									
Insulin Dose									
Grams Carb									
Activity									

Date:	Breakfast	Snack	Lunch	Snack	Dinner	Snack	Bedtime	Night	Notes
Blood Sugar									
Insulin Dose									
Grams Carb									
Activity									

Date:	Breakfast	Snack	Lunch	Snack	Dinner	Snack	Bedtime	Night	Notes
Blood Sugar									
Insulin Dose									
Grams Carb									
Activity									

Date:	Breakfast	Snack	Lunch	Snack	Dinner	Snack	Bedtime	Night	Notes
Blood Sugar									
Insulin Dose									
Grams Carb									
Activity									

Date:	Breakfast	Snack	Lunch	Snack	Dinner	Snack	Bedtime	Night	Notes
Blood Sugar									
Insulin Dose									
Grams Carb									
Activity									

Date:	Breakfast	Snack	Lunch	Snack	Dinner	Snack	Bedtime	Night	Notes
Blood Sugar									
Insulin Dose									
Grams Carb									
Activity									

Weekly Diabetes Record

Name: _____

Date:	Breakfast	Snack	Lunch	Snack	Dinner	Snack	Bedtime	Night	Notes
Blood Sugar									
Insulin Dose									
Grams Carb									
Activity									

Date:	Breakfast	Snack	Lunch	Snack	Dinner	Snack	Bedtime	Night	Notes
Blood Sugar									
Insulin Dose									
Grams Carb									
Activity									

Date:	Breakfast	Snack	Lunch	Snack	Dinner	Snack	Bedtime	Night	Notes
Blood Sugar									
Insulin Dose									
Grams Carb									
Activity									

Date:	Breakfast	Snack	Lunch	Snack	Dinner	Snack	Bedtime	Night	Notes
Blood Sugar									
Insulin Dose									
Grams Carb									
Activity									

Date:	Breakfast	Snack	Lunch	Snack	Dinner	Snack	Bedtime	Night	Notes
Blood Sugar									
Insulin Dose									
Grams Carb									
Activity									

Date:	Breakfast	Snack	Lunch	Snack	Dinner	Snack	Bedtime	Night	Notes
Blood Sugar									
Insulin Dose									
Grams Carb									
Activity									

Date:	Breakfast	Snack	Lunch	Snack	Dinner	Snack	Bedtime	Night	Notes
Blood Sugar									
Insulin Dose									
Grams Carb									
Activity									

Weekly Diabetes Record

Name: _____

Date:	Breakfast	Snack	Lunch	Snack	Dinner	Snack	Bedtime	Night	Notes
Blood Sugar									
Insulin Dose									
Grams Carb									
Activity									

Date:	Breakfast	Snack	Lunch	Snack	Dinner	Snack	Bedtime	Night	Notes
Blood Sugar									
Insulin Dose									
Grams Carb									
Activity									

Date:	Breakfast	Snack	Lunch	Snack	Dinner	Snack	Bedtime	Night	Notes
Blood Sugar									
Insulin Dose									
Grams Carb									
Activity									

Date:	Breakfast	Snack	Lunch	Snack	Dinner	Snack	Bedtime	Night	Notes
Blood Sugar									
Insulin Dose									
Grams Carb									
Activity									

Date:	Breakfast	Snack	Lunch	Snack	Dinner	Snack	Bedtime	Night	Notes
Blood Sugar									
Insulin Dose									
Grams Carb									
Activity									

Date:	Breakfast	Snack	Lunch	Snack	Dinner	Snack	Bedtime	Night	Notes
Blood Sugar									
Insulin Dose									
Grams Carb									
Activity									

Date:	Breakfast	Snack	Lunch	Snack	Dinner	Snack	Bedtime	Night	Notes
Blood Sugar									
Insulin Dose									
Grams Carb									
Activity									

Weekly Diabetes Record

Name: _____

Date:	Breakfast	Snack	Lunch	Snack	Dinner	Snack	Bedtime	Night	Notes
Blood Sugar									
Insulin Dose									
Grams Carb									
Activity									

Date:	Breakfast	Snack	Lunch	Snack	Dinner	Snack	Bedtime	Night	Notes
Blood Sugar									
Insulin Dose									
Grams Carb									
Activity									

Date:	Breakfast	Snack	Lunch	Snack	Dinner	Snack	Bedtime	Night	Notes
Blood Sugar									
Insulin Dose									
Grams Carb									
Activity									

Date:	Breakfast	Snack	Lunch	Snack	Dinner	Snack	Bedtime	Night	Notes
Blood Sugar									
Insulin Dose									
Grams Carb									
Activity									

Date:	Breakfast	Snack	Lunch	Snack	Dinner	Snack	Bedtime	Night	Notes
Blood Sugar									
Insulin Dose									
Grams Carb									
Activity									

Date:	Breakfast	Snack	Lunch	Snack	Dinner	Snack	Bedtime	Night	Notes
Blood Sugar									
Insulin Dose									
Grams Carb									
Activity									

Date:	Breakfast	Snack	Lunch	Snack	Dinner	Snack	Bedtime	Night	Notes
Blood Sugar									
Insulin Dose									
Grams Carb									
Activity									

Weekly Diabetes Record

Name: _____

Date:	Breakfast	Snack	Lunch	Snack	Dinner	Snack	Bedtime	Night	Notes
Blood Sugar									
Insulin Dose									
Grams Carb									
Activity									

Date:	Breakfast	Snack	Lunch	Snack	Dinner	Snack	Bedtime	Night	Notes
Blood Sugar									
Insulin Dose									
Grams Carb									
Activity									

Date:	Breakfast	Snack	Lunch	Snack	Dinner	Snack	Bedtime	Night	Notes
Blood Sugar									
Insulin Dose									
Grams Carb									
Activity									

Date:	Breakfast	Snack	Lunch	Snack	Dinner	Snack	Bedtime	Night	Notes
Blood Sugar									
Insulin Dose									
Grams Carb									
Activity									

Date:	Breakfast	Snack	Lunch	Snack	Dinner	Snack	Bedtime	Night	Notes
Blood Sugar									
Insulin Dose									
Grams Carb									
Activity									

Date:	Breakfast	Snack	Lunch	Snack	Dinner	Snack	Bedtime	Night	Notes
Blood Sugar									
Insulin Dose									
Grams Carb									
Activity									

Date:	Breakfast	Snack	Lunch	Snack	Dinner	Snack	Bedtime	Night	Notes
Blood Sugar									
Insulin Dose									
Grams Carb									
Activity									

Weekly Diabetes Record

Name: _____

Date:	Breakfast	Snack	Lunch	Snack	Dinner	Snack	Bedtime	Night	Notes
Blood Sugar									
Insulin Dose									
Grams Carb									
Activity									

Date:	Breakfast	Snack	Lunch	Snack	Dinner	Snack	Bedtime	Night	Notes
Blood Sugar									
Insulin Dose									
Grams Carb									
Activity									

Date:	Breakfast	Snack	Lunch	Snack	Dinner	Snack	Bedtime	Night	Notes
Blood Sugar									
Insulin Dose									
Grams Carb									
Activity									

Date:	Breakfast	Snack	Lunch	Snack	Dinner	Snack	Bedtime	Night	Notes
Blood Sugar									
Insulin Dose									
Grams Carb									
Activity									

Date:	Breakfast	Snack	Lunch	Snack	Dinner	Snack	Bedtime	Night	Notes
Blood Sugar									
Insulin Dose									
Grams Carb									
Activity									

Date:	Breakfast	Snack	Lunch	Snack	Dinner	Snack	Bedtime	Night	Notes
Blood Sugar									
Insulin Dose									
Grams Carb									
Activity									

Date:	Breakfast	Snack	Lunch	Snack	Dinner	Snack	Bedtime	Night	Notes
Blood Sugar									
Insulin Dose									
Grams Carb									
Activity									

Weekly Diabetes Record

Name: _____

Date:	Breakfast	Snack	Lunch	Snack	Dinner	Snack	Bedtime	Night	Notes
Blood Sugar									
Insulin Dose									
Grams Carb									
Activity									

Date:	Breakfast	Snack	Lunch	Snack	Dinner	Snack	Bedtime	Night	Notes
Blood Sugar									
Insulin Dose									
Grams Carb									
Activity									

Date:	Breakfast	Snack	Lunch	Snack	Dinner	Snack	Bedtime	Night	Notes
Blood Sugar									
Insulin Dose									
Grams Carb									
Activity									

Date:	Breakfast	Snack	Lunch	Snack	Dinner	Snack	Bedtime	Night	Notes
Blood Sugar									
Insulin Dose									
Grams Carb									
Activity									

Date:	Breakfast	Snack	Lunch	Snack	Dinner	Snack	Bedtime	Night	Notes
Blood Sugar									
Insulin Dose									
Grams Carb									
Activity									

Date:	Breakfast	Snack	Lunch	Snack	Dinner	Snack	Bedtime	Night	Notes
Blood Sugar									
Insulin Dose									
Grams Carb									
Activity									

Date:	Breakfast	Snack	Lunch	Snack	Dinner	Snack	Bedtime	Night	Notes
Blood Sugar									
Insulin Dose									
Grams Carb									
Activity									

Weekly Diabetes Record

Name: _____

Date:	Breakfast	Snack	Lunch	Snack	Dinner	Snack	Bedtime	Night	Notes
Blood Sugar									
Insulin Dose									
Grams Carb									
Activity									

Date:	Breakfast	Snack	Lunch	Snack	Dinner	Snack	Bedtime	Night	Notes
Blood Sugar									
Insulin Dose									
Grams Carb									
Activity									

Date:	Breakfast	Snack	Lunch	Snack	Dinner	Snack	Bedtime	Night	Notes
Blood Sugar									
Insulin Dose									
Grams Carb									
Activity									

Date:	Breakfast	Snack	Lunch	Snack	Dinner	Snack	Bedtime	Night	Notes
Blood Sugar									
Insulin Dose									
Grams Carb									
Activity									

Date:	Breakfast	Snack	Lunch	Snack	Dinner	Snack	Bedtime	Night	Notes
Blood Sugar									
Insulin Dose									
Grams Carb									
Activity									

Date:	Breakfast	Snack	Lunch	Snack	Dinner	Snack	Bedtime	Night	Notes
Blood Sugar									
Insulin Dose									
Grams Carb									
Activity									

Date:	Breakfast	Snack	Lunch	Snack	Dinner	Snack	Bedtime	Night	Notes
Blood Sugar									
Insulin Dose									
Grams Carb									
Activity									

Weekly Diabetes Record

Name: _____

Date:	Breakfast	Snack	Lunch	Snack	Dinner	Snack	Bedtime	Night	Notes
Blood Sugar									
Insulin Dose									
Grams Carb									
Activity									

Date:	Breakfast	Snack	Lunch	Snack	Dinner	Snack	Bedtime	Night	Notes
Blood Sugar									
Insulin Dose									
Grams Carb									
Activity									

Date:	Breakfast	Snack	Lunch	Snack	Dinner	Snack	Bedtime	Night	Notes
Blood Sugar									
Insulin Dose									
Grams Carb									
Activity									

Date:	Breakfast	Snack	Lunch	Snack	Dinner	Snack	Bedtime	Night	Notes
Blood Sugar									
Insulin Dose									
Grams Carb									
Activity									

Date:	Breakfast	Snack	Lunch	Snack	Dinner	Snack	Bedtime	Night	Notes
Blood Sugar									
Insulin Dose									
Grams Carb									
Activity									

Date:	Breakfast	Snack	Lunch	Snack	Dinner	Snack	Bedtime	Night	Notes
Blood Sugar									
Insulin Dose									
Grams Carb									
Activity									

Date:	Breakfast	Snack	Lunch	Snack	Dinner	Snack	Bedtime	Night	Notes
Blood Sugar									
Insulin Dose									
Grams Carb									
Activity									

Weekly Diabetes Record

Name: _____

Date:	Breakfast	Snack	Lunch	Snack	Dinner	Snack	Bedtime	Night	Notes
Blood Sugar									
Insulin Dose									
Grams Carb									
Activity									

Date:	Breakfast	Snack	Lunch	Snack	Dinner	Snack	Bedtime	Night	Notes
Blood Sugar									
Insulin Dose									
Grams Carb									
Activity									

Date:	Breakfast	Snack	Lunch	Snack	Dinner	Snack	Bedtime	Night	Notes
Blood Sugar									
Insulin Dose									
Grams Carb									
Activity									

Date:	Breakfast	Snack	Lunch	Snack	Dinner	Snack	Bedtime	Night	Notes
Blood Sugar									
Insulin Dose									
Grams Carb									
Activity									

Date:	Breakfast	Snack	Lunch	Snack	Dinner	Snack	Bedtime	Night	Notes
Blood Sugar									
Insulin Dose									
Grams Carb									
Activity									

Date:	Breakfast	Snack	Lunch	Snack	Dinner	Snack	Bedtime	Night	Notes
Blood Sugar									
Insulin Dose									
Grams Carb									
Activity									

Date:	Breakfast	Snack	Lunch	Snack	Dinner	Snack	Bedtime	Night	Notes
Blood Sugar									
Insulin Dose									
Grams Carb									
Activity									

Weekly Diabetes Record

Name: _____

Date:	Breakfast	Snack	Lunch	Snack	Dinner	Snack	Bedtime	Night	Notes
Blood Sugar									
Insulin Dose									
Grams Carb									
Activity									

Date:	Breakfast	Snack	Lunch	Snack	Dinner	Snack	Bedtime	Night	Notes
Blood Sugar									
Insulin Dose									
Grams Carb									
Activity									

Date:	Breakfast	Snack	Lunch	Snack	Dinner	Snack	Bedtime	Night	Notes
Blood Sugar									
Insulin Dose									
Grams Carb									
Activity									

Date:	Breakfast	Snack	Lunch	Snack	Dinner	Snack	Bedtime	Night	Notes
Blood Sugar									
Insulin Dose									
Grams Carb									
Activity									

Date:	Breakfast	Snack	Lunch	Snack	Dinner	Snack	Bedtime	Night	Notes
Blood Sugar									
Insulin Dose									
Grams Carb									
Activity									

Date:	Breakfast	Snack	Lunch	Snack	Dinner	Snack	Bedtime	Night	Notes
Blood Sugar									
Insulin Dose									
Grams Carb									
Activity									

Date:	Breakfast	Snack	Lunch	Snack	Dinner	Snack	Bedtime	Night	Notes
Blood Sugar									
Insulin Dose									
Grams Carb									
Activity									

Weekly Diabetes Record

Name: _____

Date:	Breakfast	Snack	Lunch	Snack	Dinner	Snack	Bedtime	Night	Notes
Blood Sugar									
Insulin Dose									
Grams Carb									
Activity									

Date:	Breakfast	Snack	Lunch	Snack	Dinner	Snack	Bedtime	Night	Notes
Blood Sugar									
Insulin Dose									
Grams Carb									
Activity									

Date:	Breakfast	Snack	Lunch	Snack	Dinner	Snack	Bedtime	Night	Notes
Blood Sugar									
Insulin Dose									
Grams Carb									
Activity									

Date:	Breakfast	Snack	Lunch	Snack	Dinner	Snack	Bedtime	Night	Notes
Blood Sugar									
Insulin Dose									
Grams Carb									
Activity									

Date:	Breakfast	Snack	Lunch	Snack	Dinner	Snack	Bedtime	Night	Notes
Blood Sugar									
Insulin Dose									
Grams Carb									
Activity									

Date:	Breakfast	Snack	Lunch	Snack	Dinner	Snack	Bedtime	Night	Notes
Blood Sugar									
Insulin Dose									
Grams Carb									
Activity									

Date:	Breakfast	Snack	Lunch	Snack	Dinner	Snack	Bedtime	Night	Notes
Blood Sugar									
Insulin Dose									
Grams Carb									
Activity									

Weekly Diabetes Record

Name: _____

Date:	Breakfast	Snack	Lunch	Snack	Dinner	Snack	Bedtime	Night	Notes
Blood Sugar									
Insulin Dose									
Grams Carb									
Activity									

Date:	Breakfast	Snack	Lunch	Snack	Dinner	Snack	Bedtime	Night	Notes
Blood Sugar									
Insulin Dose									
Grams Carb									
Activity									

Date:	Breakfast	Snack	Lunch	Snack	Dinner	Snack	Bedtime	Night	Notes
Blood Sugar									
Insulin Dose									
Grams Carb									
Activity									

Date:	Breakfast	Snack	Lunch	Snack	Dinner	Snack	Bedtime	Night	Notes
Blood Sugar									
Insulin Dose									
Grams Carb									
Activity									

Date:	Breakfast	Snack	Lunch	Snack	Dinner	Snack	Bedtime	Night	Notes
Blood Sugar									
Insulin Dose									
Grams Carb									
Activity									

Date:	Breakfast	Snack	Lunch	Snack	Dinner	Snack	Bedtime	Night	Notes
Blood Sugar									
Insulin Dose									
Grams Carb									
Activity									

Date:	Breakfast	Snack	Lunch	Snack	Dinner	Snack	Bedtime	Night	Notes
Blood Sugar									
Insulin Dose									
Grams Carb									
Activity									

Weekly Diabetes Record

Name: _____

Date:	Breakfast	Snack	Lunch	Snack	Dinner	Snack	Bedtime	Night	Notes
Blood Sugar									
Insulin Dose									
Grams Carb									
Activity									

Date:	Breakfast	Snack	Lunch	Snack	Dinner	Snack	Bedtime	Night	Notes
Blood Sugar									
Insulin Dose									
Grams Carb									
Activity									

Date:	Breakfast	Snack	Lunch	Snack	Dinner	Snack	Bedtime	Night	Notes
Blood Sugar									
Insulin Dose									
Grams Carb									
Activity									

Date:	Breakfast	Snack	Lunch	Snack	Dinner	Snack	Bedtime	Night	Notes
Blood Sugar									
Insulin Dose									
Grams Carb									
Activity									

Date:	Breakfast	Snack	Lunch	Snack	Dinner	Snack	Bedtime	Night	Notes
Blood Sugar									
Insulin Dose									
Grams Carb									
Activity									

Date:	Breakfast	Snack	Lunch	Snack	Dinner	Snack	Bedtime	Night	Notes
Blood Sugar									
Insulin Dose									
Grams Carb									
Activity									

Date:	Breakfast	Snack	Lunch	Snack	Dinner	Snack	Bedtime	Night	Notes
Blood Sugar									
Insulin Dose									
Grams Carb									
Activity									

Weekly Diabetes Record

Name: _____

Date:	Breakfast	Snack	Lunch	Snack	Dinner	Snack	Bedtime	Night	Notes
Blood Sugar									
Insulin Dose									
Grams Carb									
Activity									

Date:	Breakfast	Snack	Lunch	Snack	Dinner	Snack	Bedtime	Night	Notes
Blood Sugar									
Insulin Dose									
Grams Carb									
Activity									

Date:	Breakfast	Snack	Lunch	Snack	Dinner	Snack	Bedtime	Night	Notes
Blood Sugar									
Insulin Dose									
Grams Carb									
Activity									

Date:	Breakfast	Snack	Lunch	Snack	Dinner	Snack	Bedtime	Night	Notes
Blood Sugar									
Insulin Dose									
Grams Carb									
Activity									

Date:	Breakfast	Snack	Lunch	Snack	Dinner	Snack	Bedtime	Night	Notes
Blood Sugar									
Insulin Dose									
Grams Carb									
Activity									

Date:	Breakfast	Snack	Lunch	Snack	Dinner	Snack	Bedtime	Night	Notes
Blood Sugar									
Insulin Dose									
Grams Carb									
Activity									

Date:	Breakfast	Snack	Lunch	Snack	Dinner	Snack	Bedtime	Night	Notes
Blood Sugar									
Insulin Dose									
Grams Carb									
Activity									

Weekly Diabetes Record

Name: _____

Date:	Breakfast	Snack	Lunch	Snack	Dinner	Snack	Bedtime	Night	Notes
Blood Sugar									
Insulin Dose									
Grams Carb									
Activity									

Date:	Breakfast	Snack	Lunch	Snack	Dinner	Snack	Bedtime	Night	Notes
Blood Sugar									
Insulin Dose									
Grams Carb									
Activity									

Date:	Breakfast	Snack	Lunch	Snack	Dinner	Snack	Bedtime	Night	Notes
Blood Sugar									
Insulin Dose									
Grams Carb									
Activity									

Date:	Breakfast	Snack	Lunch	Snack	Dinner	Snack	Bedtime	Night	Notes
Blood Sugar									
Insulin Dose									
Grams Carb									
Activity									

Date:	Breakfast	Snack	Lunch	Snack	Dinner	Snack	Bedtime	Night	Notes
Blood Sugar									
Insulin Dose									
Grams Carb									
Activity									

Date:	Breakfast	Snack	Lunch	Snack	Dinner	Snack	Bedtime	Night	Notes
Blood Sugar									
Insulin Dose									
Grams Carb									
Activity									

Date:	Breakfast	Snack	Lunch	Snack	Dinner	Snack	Bedtime	Night	Notes
Blood Sugar									
Insulin Dose									
Grams Carb									
Activity									

Weekly Diabetes Record

Name: _____

Date:	Breakfast	Snack	Lunch	Snack	Dinner	Snack	Bedtime	Night	Notes
Blood Sugar									
Insulin Dose									
Grams Carb									
Activity									

Date:	Breakfast	Snack	Lunch	Snack	Dinner	Snack	Bedtime	Night	Notes
Blood Sugar									
Insulin Dose									
Grams Carb									
Activity									

Date:	Breakfast	Snack	Lunch	Snack	Dinner	Snack	Bedtime	Night	Notes
Blood Sugar									
Insulin Dose									
Grams Carb									
Activity									

Date:	Breakfast	Snack	Lunch	Snack	Dinner	Snack	Bedtime	Night	Notes
Blood Sugar									
Insulin Dose									
Grams Carb									
Activity									

Date:	Breakfast	Snack	Lunch	Snack	Dinner	Snack	Bedtime	Night	Notes
Blood Sugar									
Insulin Dose									
Grams Carb									
Activity									

Date:	Breakfast	Snack	Lunch	Snack	Dinner	Snack	Bedtime	Night	Notes
Blood Sugar									
Insulin Dose									
Grams Carb									
Activity									

Date:	Breakfast	Snack	Lunch	Snack	Dinner	Snack	Bedtime	Night	Notes
Blood Sugar									
Insulin Dose									
Grams Carb									
Activity									

Weekly Diabetes Record

Name: _____

Date:	Breakfast	Snack	Lunch	Snack	Dinner	Snack	Bedtime	Night	Notes
Blood Sugar									
Insulin Dose									
Grams Carb									
Activity									

Date:	Breakfast	Snack	Lunch	Snack	Dinner	Snack	Bedtime	Night	Notes
Blood Sugar									
Insulin Dose									
Grams Carb									
Activity									

Date:	Breakfast	Snack	Lunch	Snack	Dinner	Snack	Bedtime	Night	Notes
Blood Sugar									
Insulin Dose									
Grams Carb									
Activity									

Date:	Breakfast	Snack	Lunch	Snack	Dinner	Snack	Bedtime	Night	Notes
Blood Sugar									
Insulin Dose									
Grams Carb									
Activity									

Date:	Breakfast	Snack	Lunch	Snack	Dinner	Snack	Bedtime	Night	Notes
Blood Sugar									
Insulin Dose									
Grams Carb									
Activity									

Date:	Breakfast	Snack	Lunch	Snack	Dinner	Snack	Bedtime	Night	Notes
Blood Sugar									
Insulin Dose									
Grams Carb									
Activity									

Date:	Breakfast	Snack	Lunch	Snack	Dinner	Snack	Bedtime	Night	Notes
Blood Sugar									
Insulin Dose									
Grams Carb									
Activity									

Weekly Diabetes Record

Name: _____

Date:	Breakfast	Snack	Lunch	Snack	Dinner	Snack	Bedtime	Night	Notes
Blood Sugar									
Insulin Dose									
Grams Carb									
Activity									

Date:	Breakfast	Snack	Lunch	Snack	Dinner	Snack	Bedtime	Night	Notes
Blood Sugar									
Insulin Dose									
Grams Carb									
Activity									

Date:	Breakfast	Snack	Lunch	Snack	Dinner	Snack	Bedtime	Night	Notes
Blood Sugar									
Insulin Dose									
Grams Carb									
Activity									

Date:	Breakfast	Snack	Lunch	Snack	Dinner	Snack	Bedtime	Night	Notes
Blood Sugar									
Insulin Dose									
Grams Carb									
Activity									

Date:	Breakfast	Snack	Lunch	Snack	Dinner	Snack	Bedtime	Night	Notes
Blood Sugar									
Insulin Dose									
Grams Carb									
Activity									

Date:	Breakfast	Snack	Lunch	Snack	Dinner	Snack	Bedtime	Night	Notes
Blood Sugar									
Insulin Dose									
Grams Carb									
Activity									

Date:	Breakfast	Snack	Lunch	Snack	Dinner	Snack	Bedtime	Night	Notes
Blood Sugar									
Insulin Dose									
Grams Carb									
Activity									

Weekly Diabetes Record

Name: _____

Date:	Breakfast	Snack	Lunch	Snack	Dinner	Snack	Bedtime	Night	Notes
Blood Sugar									
Insulin Dose									
Grams Carb									
Activity									

Date:	Breakfast	Snack	Lunch	Snack	Dinner	Snack	Bedtime	Night	Notes
Blood Sugar									
Insulin Dose									
Grams Carb									
Activity									

Date:	Breakfast	Snack	Lunch	Snack	Dinner	Snack	Bedtime	Night	Notes
Blood Sugar									
Insulin Dose									
Grams Carb									
Activity									

Date:	Breakfast	Snack	Lunch	Snack	Dinner	Snack	Bedtime	Night	Notes
Blood Sugar									
Insulin Dose									
Grams Carb									
Activity									

Date:	Breakfast	Snack	Lunch	Snack	Dinner	Snack	Bedtime	Night	Notes
Blood Sugar									
Insulin Dose									
Grams Carb									
Activity									

Date:	Breakfast	Snack	Lunch	Snack	Dinner	Snack	Bedtime	Night	Notes
Blood Sugar									
Insulin Dose									
Grams Carb									
Activity									

Date:	Breakfast	Snack	Lunch	Snack	Dinner	Snack	Bedtime	Night	Notes
Blood Sugar									
Insulin Dose									
Grams Carb									
Activity									

Weekly Diabetes Record

Name: _____

Date:	Breakfast	Snack	Lunch	Snack	Dinner	Snack	Bedtime	Night	Notes
Blood Sugar									
Insulin Dose									
Grams Carb									
Activity									

Date:	Breakfast	Snack	Lunch	Snack	Dinner	Snack	Bedtime	Night	Notes
Blood Sugar									
Insulin Dose									
Grams Carb									
Activity									

Date:	Breakfast	Snack	Lunch	Snack	Dinner	Snack	Bedtime	Night	Notes
Blood Sugar									
Insulin Dose									
Grams Carb									
Activity									

Date:	Breakfast	Snack	Lunch	Snack	Dinner	Snack	Bedtime	Night	Notes
Blood Sugar									
Insulin Dose									
Grams Carb									
Activity									

Date:	Breakfast	Snack	Lunch	Snack	Dinner	Snack	Bedtime	Night	Notes
Blood Sugar									
Insulin Dose									
Grams Carb									
Activity									

Date:	Breakfast	Snack	Lunch	Snack	Dinner	Snack	Bedtime	Night	Notes
Blood Sugar									
Insulin Dose									
Grams Carb									
Activity									

Date:	Breakfast	Snack	Lunch	Snack	Dinner	Snack	Bedtime	Night	Notes
Blood Sugar									
Insulin Dose									
Grams Carb									
Activity									

Weekly Diabetes Record

Name: _____

Date:	Breakfast	Snack	Lunch	Snack	Dinner	Snack	Bedtime	Night	Notes
Blood Sugar									
Insulin Dose									
Grams Carb									
Activity									

Date:	Breakfast	Snack	Lunch	Snack	Dinner	Snack	Bedtime	Night	Notes
Blood Sugar									
Insulin Dose									
Grams Carb									
Activity									

Date:	Breakfast	Snack	Lunch	Snack	Dinner	Snack	Bedtime	Night	Notes
Blood Sugar									
Insulin Dose									
Grams Carb									
Activity									

Date:	Breakfast	Snack	Lunch	Snack	Dinner	Snack	Bedtime	Night	Notes
Blood Sugar									
Insulin Dose									
Grams Carb									
Activity									

Date:	Breakfast	Snack	Lunch	Snack	Dinner	Snack	Bedtime	Night	Notes
Blood Sugar									
Insulin Dose									
Grams Carb									
Activity									

Date:	Breakfast	Snack	Lunch	Snack	Dinner	Snack	Bedtime	Night	Notes
Blood Sugar									
Insulin Dose									
Grams Carb									
Activity									

Date:	Breakfast	Snack	Lunch	Snack	Dinner	Snack	Bedtime	Night	Notes
Blood Sugar									
Insulin Dose									
Grams Carb									
Activity									

Weekly Diabetes Record

Name: _____

Date:	Breakfast	Snack	Lunch	Snack	Dinner	Snack	Bedtime	Night	Notes
Blood Sugar									
Insulin Dose									
Grams Carb									
Activity									

Date:	Breakfast	Snack	Lunch	Snack	Dinner	Snack	Bedtime	Night	Notes
Blood Sugar									
Insulin Dose									
Grams Carb									
Activity									

Date:	Breakfast	Snack	Lunch	Snack	Dinner	Snack	Bedtime	Night	Notes
Blood Sugar									
Insulin Dose									
Grams Carb									
Activity									

Date:	Breakfast	Snack	Lunch	Snack	Dinner	Snack	Bedtime	Night	Notes
Blood Sugar									
Insulin Dose									
Grams Carb									
Activity									

Date:	Breakfast	Snack	Lunch	Snack	Dinner	Snack	Bedtime	Night	Notes
Blood Sugar									
Insulin Dose									
Grams Carb									
Activity									

Date:	Breakfast	Snack	Lunch	Snack	Dinner	Snack	Bedtime	Night	Notes
Blood Sugar									
Insulin Dose									
Grams Carb									
Activity									

Date:	Breakfast	Snack	Lunch	Snack	Dinner	Snack	Bedtime	Night	Notes
Blood Sugar									
Insulin Dose									
Grams Carb									
Activity									

Weekly Diabetes Record

Name: _____

Date:	Breakfast	Snack	Lunch	Snack	Dinner	Snack	Bedtime	Night	Notes
Blood Sugar									
Insulin Dose									
Grams Carb									
Activity									

Date:	Breakfast	Snack	Lunch	Snack	Dinner	Snack	Bedtime	Night	Notes
Blood Sugar									
Insulin Dose									
Grams Carb									
Activity									

Date:	Breakfast	Snack	Lunch	Snack	Dinner	Snack	Bedtime	Night	Notes
Blood Sugar									
Insulin Dose									
Grams Carb									
Activity									

Date:	Breakfast	Snack	Lunch	Snack	Dinner	Snack	Bedtime	Night	Notes
Blood Sugar									
Insulin Dose									
Grams Carb									
Activity									

Date:	Breakfast	Snack	Lunch	Snack	Dinner	Snack	Bedtime	Night	Notes
Blood Sugar									
Insulin Dose									
Grams Carb									
Activity									

Date:	Breakfast	Snack	Lunch	Snack	Dinner	Snack	Bedtime	Night	Notes
Blood Sugar									
Insulin Dose									
Grams Carb									
Activity									

Date:	Breakfast	Snack	Lunch	Snack	Dinner	Snack	Bedtime	Night	Notes
Blood Sugar									
Insulin Dose									
Grams Carb									
Activity									

Weekly Diabetes Record

Name: _____

Date:	Breakfast	Snack	Lunch	Snack	Dinner	Snack	Bedtime	Night	Notes
Blood Sugar									
Insulin Dose									
Grams Carb									
Activity									

Date:	Breakfast	Snack	Lunch	Snack	Dinner	Snack	Bedtime	Night	Notes
Blood Sugar									
Insulin Dose									
Grams Carb									
Activity									

Date:	Breakfast	Snack	Lunch	Snack	Dinner	Snack	Bedtime	Night	Notes
Blood Sugar									
Insulin Dose									
Grams Carb									
Activity									

Date:	Breakfast	Snack	Lunch	Snack	Dinner	Snack	Bedtime	Night	Notes
Blood Sugar									
Insulin Dose									
Grams Carb									
Activity									

Date:	Breakfast	Snack	Lunch	Snack	Dinner	Snack	Bedtime	Night	Notes
Blood Sugar									
Insulin Dose									
Grams Carb									
Activity									

Date:	Breakfast	Snack	Lunch	Snack	Dinner	Snack	Bedtime	Night	Notes
Blood Sugar									
Insulin Dose									
Grams Carb									
Activity									

Date:	Breakfast	Snack	Lunch	Snack	Dinner	Snack	Bedtime	Night	Notes
Blood Sugar									
Insulin Dose									
Grams Carb									
Activity									

Weekly Diabetes Record

Name: _____

Date:	Breakfast	Snack	Lunch	Snack	Dinner	Snack	Bedtime	Night	Notes
Blood Sugar									
Insulin Dose									
Grams Carb									
Activity									

Date:	Breakfast	Snack	Lunch	Snack	Dinner	Snack	Bedtime	Night	Notes
Blood Sugar									
Insulin Dose									
Grams Carb									
Activity									

Date:	Breakfast	Snack	Lunch	Snack	Dinner	Snack	Bedtime	Night	Notes
Blood Sugar									
Insulin Dose									
Grams Carb									
Activity									

Date:	Breakfast	Snack	Lunch	Snack	Dinner	Snack	Bedtime	Night	Notes
Blood Sugar									
Insulin Dose									
Grams Carb									
Activity									

Date:	Breakfast	Snack	Lunch	Snack	Dinner	Snack	Bedtime	Night	Notes
Blood Sugar									
Insulin Dose									
Grams Carb									
Activity									

Date:	Breakfast	Snack	Lunch	Snack	Dinner	Snack	Bedtime	Night	Notes
Blood Sugar									
Insulin Dose									
Grams Carb									
Activity									

Date:	Breakfast	Snack	Lunch	Snack	Dinner	Snack	Bedtime	Night	Notes
Blood Sugar									
Insulin Dose									
Grams Carb									
Activity									

Weekly Diabetes Record

Name: _____

Date:	Breakfast	Snack	Lunch	Snack	Dinner	Snack	Bedtime	Night	Notes
Blood Sugar									
Insulin Dose									
Grams Carb									
Activity									

Date:	Breakfast	Snack	Lunch	Snack	Dinner	Snack	Bedtime	Night	Notes
Blood Sugar									
Insulin Dose									
Grams Carb									
Activity									

Date:	Breakfast	Snack	Lunch	Snack	Dinner	Snack	Bedtime	Night	Notes
Blood Sugar									
Insulin Dose									
Grams Carb									
Activity									

Date:	Breakfast	Snack	Lunch	Snack	Dinner	Snack	Bedtime	Night	Notes
Blood Sugar									
Insulin Dose									
Grams Carb									
Activity									

Date:	Breakfast	Snack	Lunch	Snack	Dinner	Snack	Bedtime	Night	Notes
Blood Sugar									
Insulin Dose									
Grams Carb									
Activity									

Date:	Breakfast	Snack	Lunch	Snack	Dinner	Snack	Bedtime	Night	Notes
Blood Sugar									
Insulin Dose									
Grams Carb									
Activity									

Date:	Breakfast	Snack	Lunch	Snack	Dinner	Snack	Bedtime	Night	Notes
Blood Sugar									
Insulin Dose									
Grams Carb									
Activity									

Weekly Diabetes Record

Name: _____

Date:	Breakfast	Snack	Lunch	Snack	Dinner	Snack	Bedtime	Night	Notes
Blood Sugar									
Insulin Dose									
Grams Carb									
Activity									

Date:	Breakfast	Snack	Lunch	Snack	Dinner	Snack	Bedtime	Night	Notes
Blood Sugar									
Insulin Dose									
Grams Carb									
Activity									

Date:	Breakfast	Snack	Lunch	Snack	Dinner	Snack	Bedtime	Night	Notes
Blood Sugar									
Insulin Dose									
Grams Carb									
Activity									

Date:	Breakfast	Snack	Lunch	Snack	Dinner	Snack	Bedtime	Night	Notes
Blood Sugar									
Insulin Dose									
Grams Carb									
Activity									

Date:	Breakfast	Snack	Lunch	Snack	Dinner	Snack	Bedtime	Night	Notes
Blood Sugar									
Insulin Dose									
Grams Carb									
Activity									

Date:	Breakfast	Snack	Lunch	Snack	Dinner	Snack	Bedtime	Night	Notes
Blood Sugar									
Insulin Dose									
Grams Carb									
Activity									

Date:	Breakfast	Snack	Lunch	Snack	Dinner	Snack	Bedtime	Night	Notes
Blood Sugar									
Insulin Dose									
Grams Carb									
Activity									

Weekly Diabetes Record

Name: _____

Date:	Breakfast	Snack	Lunch	Snack	Dinner	Snack	Bedtime	Night	Notes
Blood Sugar									
Insulin Dose									
Grams Carb									
Activity									

Date:	Breakfast	Snack	Lunch	Snack	Dinner	Snack	Bedtime	Night	Notes
Blood Sugar									
Insulin Dose									
Grams Carb									
Activity									

Date:	Breakfast	Snack	Lunch	Snack	Dinner	Snack	Bedtime	Night	Notes
Blood Sugar									
Insulin Dose									
Grams Carb									
Activity									

Date:	Breakfast	Snack	Lunch	Snack	Dinner	Snack	Bedtime	Night	Notes
Blood Sugar									
Insulin Dose									
Grams Carb									
Activity									

Date:	Breakfast	Snack	Lunch	Snack	Dinner	Snack	Bedtime	Night	Notes
Blood Sugar									
Insulin Dose									
Grams Carb									
Activity									

Date:	Breakfast	Snack	Lunch	Snack	Dinner	Snack	Bedtime	Night	Notes
Blood Sugar									
Insulin Dose									
Grams Carb									
Activity									

Date:	Breakfast	Snack	Lunch	Snack	Dinner	Snack	Bedtime	Night	Notes
Blood Sugar									
Insulin Dose									
Grams Carb									
Activity									

Weekly Diabetes Record

Name: _____

Date:	Breakfast	Snack	Lunch	Snack	Dinner	Snack	Bedtime	Night	Notes
Blood Sugar									
Insulin Dose									
Grams Carb									
Activity									

Date:	Breakfast	Snack	Lunch	Snack	Dinner	Snack	Bedtime	Night	Notes
Blood Sugar									
Insulin Dose									
Grams Carb									
Activity									

Date:	Breakfast	Snack	Lunch	Snack	Dinner	Snack	Bedtime	Night	Notes
Blood Sugar									
Insulin Dose									
Grams Carb									
Activity									

Date:	Breakfast	Snack	Lunch	Snack	Dinner	Snack	Bedtime	Night	Notes
Blood Sugar									
Insulin Dose									
Grams Carb									
Activity									

Date:	Breakfast	Snack	Lunch	Snack	Dinner	Snack	Bedtime	Night	Notes
Blood Sugar									
Insulin Dose									
Grams Carb									
Activity									

Date:	Breakfast	Snack	Lunch	Snack	Dinner	Snack	Bedtime	Night	Notes
Blood Sugar									
Insulin Dose									
Grams Carb									
Activity									

Date:	Breakfast	Snack	Lunch	Snack	Dinner	Snack	Bedtime	Night	Notes
Blood Sugar									
Insulin Dose									
Grams Carb									
Activity									

Weekly Diabetes Record

Name: _____

Date:	Breakfast	Snack	Lunch	Snack	Dinner	Snack	Bedtime	Night	Notes
Blood Sugar									
Insulin Dose									
Grams Carb									
Activity									

Date:	Breakfast	Snack	Lunch	Snack	Dinner	Snack	Bedtime	Night	Notes
Blood Sugar									
Insulin Dose									
Grams Carb									
Activity									

Date:	Breakfast	Snack	Lunch	Snack	Dinner	Snack	Bedtime	Night	Notes
Blood Sugar									
Insulin Dose									
Grams Carb									
Activity									

Date:	Breakfast	Snack	Lunch	Snack	Dinner	Snack	Bedtime	Night	Notes
Blood Sugar									
Insulin Dose									
Grams Carb									
Activity									

Date:	Breakfast	Snack	Lunch	Snack	Dinner	Snack	Bedtime	Night	Notes
Blood Sugar									
Insulin Dose									
Grams Carb									
Activity									

Date:	Breakfast	Snack	Lunch	Snack	Dinner	Snack	Bedtime	Night	Notes
Blood Sugar									
Insulin Dose									
Grams Carb									
Activity									

Date:	Breakfast	Snack	Lunch	Snack	Dinner	Snack	Bedtime	Night	Notes
Blood Sugar									
Insulin Dose									
Grams Carb									
Activity									

Weekly Diabetes Record

Name: _____

Date:	Breakfast	Snack	Lunch	Snack	Dinner	Snack	Bedtime	Night	Notes
Blood Sugar									
Insulin Dose									
Grams Carb									
Activity									

Date:	Breakfast	Snack	Lunch	Snack	Dinner	Snack	Bedtime	Night	Notes
Blood Sugar									
Insulin Dose									
Grams Carb									
Activity									

Date:	Breakfast	Snack	Lunch	Snack	Dinner	Snack	Bedtime	Night	Notes
Blood Sugar									
Insulin Dose									
Grams Carb									
Activity									

Date:	Breakfast	Snack	Lunch	Snack	Dinner	Snack	Bedtime	Night	Notes
Blood Sugar									
Insulin Dose									
Grams Carb									
Activity									

Date:	Breakfast	Snack	Lunch	Snack	Dinner	Snack	Bedtime	Night	Notes
Blood Sugar									
Insulin Dose									
Grams Carb									
Activity									

Date:	Breakfast	Snack	Lunch	Snack	Dinner	Snack	Bedtime	Night	Notes
Blood Sugar									
Insulin Dose									
Grams Carb									
Activity									

Date:	Breakfast	Snack	Lunch	Snack	Dinner	Snack	Bedtime	Night	Notes
Blood Sugar									
Insulin Dose									
Grams Carb									
Activity									

Weekly Diabetes Record

Name: _____

Date:	Breakfast	Snack	Lunch	Snack	Dinner	Snack	Bedtime	Night	Notes
Blood Sugar									
Insulin Dose									
Grams Carb									
Activity									

Date:	Breakfast	Snack	Lunch	Snack	Dinner	Snack	Bedtime	Night	Notes
Blood Sugar									
Insulin Dose									
Grams Carb									
Activity									

Date:	Breakfast	Snack	Lunch	Snack	Dinner	Snack	Bedtime	Night	Notes
Blood Sugar									
Insulin Dose									
Grams Carb									
Activity									

Date:	Breakfast	Snack	Lunch	Snack	Dinner	Snack	Bedtime	Night	Notes
Blood Sugar									
Insulin Dose									
Grams Carb									
Activity									

Date:	Breakfast	Snack	Lunch	Snack	Dinner	Snack	Bedtime	Night	Notes
Blood Sugar									
Insulin Dose									
Grams Carb									
Activity									

Date:	Breakfast	Snack	Lunch	Snack	Dinner	Snack	Bedtime	Night	Notes
Blood Sugar									
Insulin Dose									
Grams Carb									
Activity									

Date:	Breakfast	Snack	Lunch	Snack	Dinner	Snack	Bedtime	Night	Notes
Blood Sugar									
Insulin Dose									
Grams Carb									
Activity									

Weekly Diabetes Record

Name: _____

Date:	Breakfast	Snack	Lunch	Snack	Dinner	Snack	Bedtime	Night	Notes
Blood Sugar									
Insulin Dose									
Grams Carb									
Activity									

Date:	Breakfast	Snack	Lunch	Snack	Dinner	Snack	Bedtime	Night	Notes
Blood Sugar									
Insulin Dose									
Grams Carb									
Activity									

Date:	Breakfast	Snack	Lunch	Snack	Dinner	Snack	Bedtime	Night	Notes
Blood Sugar									
Insulin Dose									
Grams Carb									
Activity									

Date:	Breakfast	Snack	Lunch	Snack	Dinner	Snack	Bedtime	Night	Notes
Blood Sugar									
Insulin Dose									
Grams Carb									
Activity									

Date:	Breakfast	Snack	Lunch	Snack	Dinner	Snack	Bedtime	Night	Notes
Blood Sugar									
Insulin Dose									
Grams Carb									
Activity									

Date:	Breakfast	Snack	Lunch	Snack	Dinner	Snack	Bedtime	Night	Notes
Blood Sugar									
Insulin Dose									
Grams Carb									
Activity									

Date:	Breakfast	Snack	Lunch	Snack	Dinner	Snack	Bedtime	Night	Notes
Blood Sugar									
Insulin Dose									
Grams Carb									
Activity									

Weekly Diabetes Record

Name: _____

Date:	Breakfast	Snack	Lunch	Snack	Dinner	Snack	Bedtime	Night	Notes
Blood Sugar									
Insulin Dose									
Grams Carb									
Activity									

Date:	Breakfast	Snack	Lunch	Snack	Dinner	Snack	Bedtime	Night	Notes
Blood Sugar									
Insulin Dose									
Grams Carb									
Activity									

Date:	Breakfast	Snack	Lunch	Snack	Dinner	Snack	Bedtime	Night	Notes
Blood Sugar									
Insulin Dose									
Grams Carb									
Activity									

Date:	Breakfast	Snack	Lunch	Snack	Dinner	Snack	Bedtime	Night	Notes
Blood Sugar									
Insulin Dose									
Grams Carb									
Activity									

Date:	Breakfast	Snack	Lunch	Snack	Dinner	Snack	Bedtime	Night	Notes
Blood Sugar									
Insulin Dose									
Grams Carb									
Activity									

Date:	Breakfast	Snack	Lunch	Snack	Dinner	Snack	Bedtime	Night	Notes
Blood Sugar									
Insulin Dose									
Grams Carb									
Activity									

Date:	Breakfast	Snack	Lunch	Snack	Dinner	Snack	Bedtime	Night	Notes
Blood Sugar									
Insulin Dose									
Grams Carb									
Activity									

Weekly Diabetes Record

Name: _____

Date:	Breakfast	Snack	Lunch	Snack	Dinner	Snack	Bedtime	Night	Notes
Blood Sugar									
Insulin Dose									
Grams Carb									
Activity									

Date:	Breakfast	Snack	Lunch	Snack	Dinner	Snack	Bedtime	Night	Notes
Blood Sugar									
Insulin Dose									
Grams Carb									
Activity									

Date:	Breakfast	Snack	Lunch	Snack	Dinner	Snack	Bedtime	Night	Notes
Blood Sugar									
Insulin Dose									
Grams Carb									
Activity									

Date:	Breakfast	Snack	Lunch	Snack	Dinner	Snack	Bedtime	Night	Notes
Blood Sugar									
Insulin Dose									
Grams Carb									
Activity									

Date:	Breakfast	Snack	Lunch	Snack	Dinner	Snack	Bedtime	Night	Notes
Blood Sugar									
Insulin Dose									
Grams Carb									
Activity									

Date:	Breakfast	Snack	Lunch	Snack	Dinner	Snack	Bedtime	Night	Notes
Blood Sugar									
Insulin Dose									
Grams Carb									
Activity									

Date:	Breakfast	Snack	Lunch	Snack	Dinner	Snack	Bedtime	Night	Notes
Blood Sugar									
Insulin Dose									
Grams Carb									
Activity									

Weekly Diabetes Record

Name: _____

Date:	Breakfast	Snack	Lunch	Snack	Dinner	Snack	Bedtime	Night	Notes
Blood Sugar									
Insulin Dose									
Grams Carb									
Activity									

Date:	Breakfast	Snack	Lunch	Snack	Dinner	Snack	Bedtime	Night	Notes
Blood Sugar									
Insulin Dose									
Grams Carb									
Activity									

Date:	Breakfast	Snack	Lunch	Snack	Dinner	Snack	Bedtime	Night	Notes
Blood Sugar									
Insulin Dose									
Grams Carb									
Activity									

Date:	Breakfast	Snack	Lunch	Snack	Dinner	Snack	Bedtime	Night	Notes
Blood Sugar									
Insulin Dose									
Grams Carb									
Activity									

Date:	Breakfast	Snack	Lunch	Snack	Dinner	Snack	Bedtime	Night	Notes
Blood Sugar									
Insulin Dose									
Grams Carb									
Activity									

Date:	Breakfast	Snack	Lunch	Snack	Dinner	Snack	Bedtime	Night	Notes
Blood Sugar									
Insulin Dose									
Grams Carb									
Activity									

Date:	Breakfast	Snack	Lunch	Snack	Dinner	Snack	Bedtime	Night	Notes
Blood Sugar									
Insulin Dose									
Grams Carb									
Activity									

Weekly Diabetes Record

Name: _____

Date:	Breakfast	Snack	Lunch	Snack	Dinner	Snack	Bedtime	Night	Notes
Blood Sugar									
Insulin Dose									
Grams Carb									
Activity									

Date:	Breakfast	Snack	Lunch	Snack	Dinner	Snack	Bedtime	Night	Notes
Blood Sugar									
Insulin Dose									
Grams Carb									
Activity									

Date:	Breakfast	Snack	Lunch	Snack	Dinner	Snack	Bedtime	Night	Notes
Blood Sugar									
Insulin Dose									
Grams Carb									
Activity									

Date:	Breakfast	Snack	Lunch	Snack	Dinner	Snack	Bedtime	Night	Notes
Blood Sugar									
Insulin Dose									
Grams Carb									
Activity									

Date:	Breakfast	Snack	Lunch	Snack	Dinner	Snack	Bedtime	Night	Notes
Blood Sugar									
Insulin Dose									
Grams Carb									
Activity									

Date:	Breakfast	Snack	Lunch	Snack	Dinner	Snack	Bedtime	Night	Notes
Blood Sugar									
Insulin Dose									
Grams Carb									
Activity									

Date:	Breakfast	Snack	Lunch	Snack	Dinner	Snack	Bedtime	Night	Notes
Blood Sugar									
Insulin Dose									
Grams Carb									
Activity									

Weekly Diabetes Record

Name: _____

Date:	Breakfast	Snack	Lunch	Snack	Dinner	Snack	Bedtime	Night	Notes
Blood Sugar									
Insulin Dose									
Grams Carb									
Activity									

Date:	Breakfast	Snack	Lunch	Snack	Dinner	Snack	Bedtime	Night	Notes
Blood Sugar									
Insulin Dose									
Grams Carb									
Activity									

Date:	Breakfast	Snack	Lunch	Snack	Dinner	Snack	Bedtime	Night	Notes
Blood Sugar									
Insulin Dose									
Grams Carb									
Activity									

Date:	Breakfast	Snack	Lunch	Snack	Dinner	Snack	Bedtime	Night	Notes
Blood Sugar									
Insulin Dose									
Grams Carb									
Activity									

Date:	Breakfast	Snack	Lunch	Snack	Dinner	Snack	Bedtime	Night	Notes
Blood Sugar									
Insulin Dose									
Grams Carb									
Activity									

Date:	Breakfast	Snack	Lunch	Snack	Dinner	Snack	Bedtime	Night	Notes
Blood Sugar									
Insulin Dose									
Grams Carb									
Activity									

Date:	Breakfast	Snack	Lunch	Snack	Dinner	Snack	Bedtime	Night	Notes
Blood Sugar									
Insulin Dose									
Grams Carb									
Activity									

Weekly Diabetes Record

Name: _____

Date:	Breakfast	Snack	Lunch	Snack	Dinner	Snack	Bedtime	Night	Notes
Blood Sugar									
Insulin Dose									
Grams Carb									
Activity									

Date:	Breakfast	Snack	Lunch	Snack	Dinner	Snack	Bedtime	Night	Notes
Blood Sugar									
Insulin Dose									
Grams Carb									
Activity									

Date:	Breakfast	Snack	Lunch	Snack	Dinner	Snack	Bedtime	Night	Notes
Blood Sugar									
Insulin Dose									
Grams Carb									
Activity									

Date:	Breakfast	Snack	Lunch	Snack	Dinner	Snack	Bedtime	Night	Notes
Blood Sugar									
Insulin Dose									
Grams Carb									
Activity									

Date:	Breakfast	Snack	Lunch	Snack	Dinner	Snack	Bedtime	Night	Notes
Blood Sugar									
Insulin Dose									
Grams Carb									
Activity									

Date:	Breakfast	Snack	Lunch	Snack	Dinner	Snack	Bedtime	Night	Notes
Blood Sugar									
Insulin Dose									
Grams Carb									
Activity									

Date:	Breakfast	Snack	Lunch	Snack	Dinner	Snack	Bedtime	Night	Notes
Blood Sugar									
Insulin Dose									
Grams Carb									
Activity									

Weekly Diabetes Record

Name: _____

Date:	Breakfast	Snack	Lunch	Snack	Dinner	Snack	Bedtime	Night	Notes
Blood Sugar									
Insulin Dose									
Grams Carb									
Activity									

Date:	Breakfast	Snack	Lunch	Snack	Dinner	Snack	Bedtime	Night	Notes
Blood Sugar									
Insulin Dose									
Grams Carb									
Activity									

Date:	Breakfast	Snack	Lunch	Snack	Dinner	Snack	Bedtime	Night	Notes
Blood Sugar									
Insulin Dose									
Grams Carb									
Activity									

Date:	Breakfast	Snack	Lunch	Snack	Dinner	Snack	Bedtime	Night	Notes
Blood Sugar									
Insulin Dose									
Grams Carb									
Activity									

Date:	Breakfast	Snack	Lunch	Snack	Dinner	Snack	Bedtime	Night	Notes
Blood Sugar									
Insulin Dose									
Grams Carb									
Activity									

Date:	Breakfast	Snack	Lunch	Snack	Dinner	Snack	Bedtime	Night	Notes
Blood Sugar									
Insulin Dose									
Grams Carb									
Activity									

Date:	Breakfast	Snack	Lunch	Snack	Dinner	Snack	Bedtime	Night	Notes
Blood Sugar									
Insulin Dose									
Grams Carb									
Activity									

Weekly Diabetes Record

Name: _____

Date:	Breakfast	Snack	Lunch	Snack	Dinner	Snack	Bedtime	Night	Notes
Blood Sugar									
Insulin Dose									
Grams Carb									
Activity									

Date:	Breakfast	Snack	Lunch	Snack	Dinner	Snack	Bedtime	Night	Notes
Blood Sugar									
Insulin Dose									
Grams Carb									
Activity									

Date:	Breakfast	Snack	Lunch	Snack	Dinner	Snack	Bedtime	Night	Notes
Blood Sugar									
Insulin Dose									
Grams Carb									
Activity									

Date:	Breakfast	Snack	Lunch	Snack	Dinner	Snack	Bedtime	Night	Notes
Blood Sugar									
Insulin Dose									
Grams Carb									
Activity									

Date:	Breakfast	Snack	Lunch	Snack	Dinner	Snack	Bedtime	Night	Notes
Blood Sugar									
Insulin Dose									
Grams Carb									
Activity									

Date:	Breakfast	Snack	Lunch	Snack	Dinner	Snack	Bedtime	Night	Notes
Blood Sugar									
Insulin Dose									
Grams Carb									
Activity									

Date:	Breakfast	Snack	Lunch	Snack	Dinner	Snack	Bedtime	Night	Notes
Blood Sugar									
Insulin Dose									
Grams Carb									
Activity									

Weekly Diabetes Record

Name: _____

Date:	Breakfast	Snack	Lunch	Snack	Dinner	Snack	Bedtime	Night	Notes
Blood Sugar									
Insulin Dose									
Grams Carb									
Activity									

Date:	Breakfast	Snack	Lunch	Snack	Dinner	Snack	Bedtime	Night	Notes
Blood Sugar									
Insulin Dose									
Grams Carb									
Activity									

Date:	Breakfast	Snack	Lunch	Snack	Dinner	Snack	Bedtime	Night	Notes
Blood Sugar									
Insulin Dose									
Grams Carb									
Activity									

Date:	Breakfast	Snack	Lunch	Snack	Dinner	Snack	Bedtime	Night	Notes
Blood Sugar									
Insulin Dose									
Grams Carb									
Activity									

Date:	Breakfast	Snack	Lunch	Snack	Dinner	Snack	Bedtime	Night	Notes
Blood Sugar									
Insulin Dose									
Grams Carb									
Activity									

Date:	Breakfast	Snack	Lunch	Snack	Dinner	Snack	Bedtime	Night	Notes
Blood Sugar									
Insulin Dose									
Grams Carb									
Activity									

Date:	Breakfast	Snack	Lunch	Snack	Dinner	Snack	Bedtime	Night	Notes
Blood Sugar									
Insulin Dose									
Grams Carb									
Activity									

Weekly Diabetes Record

Name: _____

Date:	Breakfast	Snack	Lunch	Snack	Dinner	Snack	Bedtime	Night	Notes
Blood Sugar									
Insulin Dose									
Grams Carb									
Activity									

Date:	Breakfast	Snack	Lunch	Snack	Dinner	Snack	Bedtime	Night	Notes
Blood Sugar									
Insulin Dose									
Grams Carb									
Activity									

Date:	Breakfast	Snack	Lunch	Snack	Dinner	Snack	Bedtime	Night	Notes
Blood Sugar									
Insulin Dose									
Grams Carb									
Activity									

Date:	Breakfast	Snack	Lunch	Snack	Dinner	Snack	Bedtime	Night	Notes
Blood Sugar									
Insulin Dose									
Grams Carb									
Activity									

Date:	Breakfast	Snack	Lunch	Snack	Dinner	Snack	Bedtime	Night	Notes
Blood Sugar									
Insulin Dose									
Grams Carb									
Activity									

Date:	Breakfast	Snack	Lunch	Snack	Dinner	Snack	Bedtime	Night	Notes
Blood Sugar									
Insulin Dose									
Grams Carb									
Activity									

Date:	Breakfast	Snack	Lunch	Snack	Dinner	Snack	Bedtime	Night	Notes
Blood Sugar									
Insulin Dose									
Grams Carb									
Activity									

Weekly Diabetes Record

Name: _____

Date:	Breakfast	Snack	Lunch	Snack	Dinner	Snack	Bedtime	Night	Notes
Blood Sugar									
Insulin Dose									
Grams Carb									
Activity									

Date:	Breakfast	Snack	Lunch	Snack	Dinner	Snack	Bedtime	Night	Notes
Blood Sugar									
Insulin Dose									
Grams Carb									
Activity									

Date:	Breakfast	Snack	Lunch	Snack	Dinner	Snack	Bedtime	Night	Notes
Blood Sugar									
Insulin Dose									
Grams Carb									
Activity									

Date:	Breakfast	Snack	Lunch	Snack	Dinner	Snack	Bedtime	Night	Notes
Blood Sugar									
Insulin Dose									
Grams Carb									
Activity									

Date:	Breakfast	Snack	Lunch	Snack	Dinner	Snack	Bedtime	Night	Notes
Blood Sugar									
Insulin Dose									
Grams Carb									
Activity									

Date:	Breakfast	Snack	Lunch	Snack	Dinner	Snack	Bedtime	Night	Notes
Blood Sugar									
Insulin Dose									
Grams Carb									
Activity									

Date:	Breakfast	Snack	Lunch	Snack	Dinner	Snack	Bedtime	Night	Notes
Blood Sugar									
Insulin Dose									
Grams Carb									
Activity									

Weekly Diabetes Record

Name: _____

Date:	Breakfast	Snack	Lunch	Snack	Dinner	Snack	Bedtime	Night	Notes
Blood Sugar									
Insulin Dose									
Grams Carb									
Activity									

Date:	Breakfast	Snack	Lunch	Snack	Dinner	Snack	Bedtime	Night	Notes
Blood Sugar									
Insulin Dose									
Grams Carb									
Activity									

Date:	Breakfast	Snack	Lunch	Snack	Dinner	Snack	Bedtime	Night	Notes
Blood Sugar									
Insulin Dose									
Grams Carb									
Activity									

Date:	Breakfast	Snack	Lunch	Snack	Dinner	Snack	Bedtime	Night	Notes
Blood Sugar									
Insulin Dose									
Grams Carb									
Activity									

Date:	Breakfast	Snack	Lunch	Snack	Dinner	Snack	Bedtime	Night	Notes
Blood Sugar									
Insulin Dose									
Grams Carb									
Activity									

Date:	Breakfast	Snack	Lunch	Snack	Dinner	Snack	Bedtime	Night	Notes
Blood Sugar									
Insulin Dose									
Grams Carb									
Activity									

Date:	Breakfast	Snack	Lunch	Snack	Dinner	Snack	Bedtime	Night	Notes
Blood Sugar									
Insulin Dose									
Grams Carb									
Activity									

Weekly Diabetes Record

Name: _____

Date:	Breakfast	Snack	Lunch	Snack	Dinner	Snack	Bedtime	Night	Notes
Blood Sugar									
Insulin Dose									
Grams Carb									
Activity									

Date:	Breakfast	Snack	Lunch	Snack	Dinner	Snack	Bedtime	Night	Notes
Blood Sugar									
Insulin Dose									
Grams Carb									
Activity									

Date:	Breakfast	Snack	Lunch	Snack	Dinner	Snack	Bedtime	Night	Notes
Blood Sugar									
Insulin Dose									
Grams Carb									
Activity									

Date:	Breakfast	Snack	Lunch	Snack	Dinner	Snack	Bedtime	Night	Notes
Blood Sugar									
Insulin Dose									
Grams Carb									
Activity									

Date:	Breakfast	Snack	Lunch	Snack	Dinner	Snack	Bedtime	Night	Notes
Blood Sugar									
Insulin Dose									
Grams Carb									
Activity									

Date:	Breakfast	Snack	Lunch	Snack	Dinner	Snack	Bedtime	Night	Notes
Blood Sugar									
Insulin Dose									
Grams Carb									
Activity									

Date:	Breakfast	Snack	Lunch	Snack	Dinner	Snack	Bedtime	Night	Notes
Blood Sugar									
Insulin Dose									
Grams Carb									
Activity									

Weekly Diabetes Record

Name: _____

Date:	Breakfast	Snack	Lunch	Snack	Dinner	Snack	Bedtime	Night	Notes
Blood Sugar									
Insulin Dose									
Grams Carb									
Activity									

Date:	Breakfast	Snack	Lunch	Snack	Dinner	Snack	Bedtime	Night	Notes
Blood Sugar									
Insulin Dose									
Grams Carb									
Activity									

Date:	Breakfast	Snack	Lunch	Snack	Dinner	Snack	Bedtime	Night	Notes
Blood Sugar									
Insulin Dose									
Grams Carb									
Activity									

Date:	Breakfast	Snack	Lunch	Snack	Dinner	Snack	Bedtime	Night	Notes
Blood Sugar									
Insulin Dose									
Grams Carb									
Activity									

Date:	Breakfast	Snack	Lunch	Snack	Dinner	Snack	Bedtime	Night	Notes
Blood Sugar									
Insulin Dose									
Grams Carb									
Activity									

Date:	Breakfast	Snack	Lunch	Snack	Dinner	Snack	Bedtime	Night	Notes
Blood Sugar									
Insulin Dose									
Grams Carb									
Activity									

Date:	Breakfast	Snack	Lunch	Snack	Dinner	Snack	Bedtime	Night	Notes
Blood Sugar									
Insulin Dose									
Grams Carb									
Activity									

Weekly Diabetes Record

Name: _____

Date:	Breakfast	Snack	Lunch	Snack	Dinner	Snack	Bedtime	Night	Notes
Blood Sugar									
Insulin Dose									
Grams Carb									
Activity									

Date:	Breakfast	Snack	Lunch	Snack	Dinner	Snack	Bedtime	Night	Notes
Blood Sugar									
Insulin Dose									
Grams Carb									
Activity									

Date:	Breakfast	Snack	Lunch	Snack	Dinner	Snack	Bedtime	Night	Notes
Blood Sugar									
Insulin Dose									
Grams Carb									
Activity									

Date:	Breakfast	Snack	Lunch	Snack	Dinner	Snack	Bedtime	Night	Notes
Blood Sugar									
Insulin Dose									
Grams Carb									
Activity									

Date:	Breakfast	Snack	Lunch	Snack	Dinner	Snack	Bedtime	Night	Notes
Blood Sugar									
Insulin Dose									
Grams Carb									
Activity									

Date:	Breakfast	Snack	Lunch	Snack	Dinner	Snack	Bedtime	Night	Notes
Blood Sugar									
Insulin Dose									
Grams Carb									
Activity									

Date:	Breakfast	Snack	Lunch	Snack	Dinner	Snack	Bedtime	Night	Notes
Blood Sugar									
Insulin Dose									
Grams Carb									
Activity									

Weekly Diabetes Record

Name: _____

Date:	Breakfast	Snack	Lunch	Snack	Dinner	Snack	Bedtime	Night	Notes
Blood Sugar									
Insulin Dose									
Grams Carb									
Activity									

Date:	Breakfast	Snack	Lunch	Snack	Dinner	Snack	Bedtime	Night	Notes
Blood Sugar									
Insulin Dose									
Grams Carb									
Activity									

Date:	Breakfast	Snack	Lunch	Snack	Dinner	Snack	Bedtime	Night	Notes
Blood Sugar									
Insulin Dose									
Grams Carb									
Activity									

Date:	Breakfast	Snack	Lunch	Snack	Dinner	Snack	Bedtime	Night	Notes
Blood Sugar									
Insulin Dose									
Grams Carb									
Activity									

Date:	Breakfast	Snack	Lunch	Snack	Dinner	Snack	Bedtime	Night	Notes
Blood Sugar									
Insulin Dose									
Grams Carb									
Activity									

Date:	Breakfast	Snack	Lunch	Snack	Dinner	Snack	Bedtime	Night	Notes
Blood Sugar									
Insulin Dose									
Grams Carb									
Activity									

Date:	Breakfast	Snack	Lunch	Snack	Dinner	Snack	Bedtime	Night	Notes
Blood Sugar									
Insulin Dose									
Grams Carb									
Activity									

Weekly Diabetes Record

Name: _____

Date:	Breakfast	Snack	Lunch	Snack	Dinner	Snack	Bedtime	Night	Notes
Blood Sugar									
Insulin Dose									
Grams Carb									
Activity									

Date:	Breakfast	Snack	Lunch	Snack	Dinner	Snack	Bedtime	Night	Notes
Blood Sugar									
Insulin Dose									
Grams Carb									
Activity									

Date:	Breakfast	Snack	Lunch	Snack	Dinner	Snack	Bedtime	Night	Notes
Blood Sugar									
Insulin Dose									
Grams Carb									
Activity									

Date:	Breakfast	Snack	Lunch	Snack	Dinner	Snack	Bedtime	Night	Notes
Blood Sugar									
Insulin Dose									
Grams Carb									
Activity									

Date:	Breakfast	Snack	Lunch	Snack	Dinner	Snack	Bedtime	Night	Notes
Blood Sugar									
Insulin Dose									
Grams Carb									
Activity									

Date:	Breakfast	Snack	Lunch	Snack	Dinner	Snack	Bedtime	Night	Notes
Blood Sugar									
Insulin Dose									
Grams Carb									
Activity									

Date:	Breakfast	Snack	Lunch	Snack	Dinner	Snack	Bedtime	Night	Notes
Blood Sugar									
Insulin Dose									
Grams Carb									
Activity									

Weekly Diabetes Record

Name: _____

Date:	Breakfast	Snack	Lunch	Snack	Dinner	Snack	Bedtime	Night	Notes
Blood Sugar									
Insulin Dose									
Grams Carb									
Activity									

Date:	Breakfast	Snack	Lunch	Snack	Dinner	Snack	Bedtime	Night	Notes
Blood Sugar									
Insulin Dose									
Grams Carb									
Activity									

Date:	Breakfast	Snack	Lunch	Snack	Dinner	Snack	Bedtime	Night	Notes
Blood Sugar									
Insulin Dose									
Grams Carb									
Activity									

Date:	Breakfast	Snack	Lunch	Snack	Dinner	Snack	Bedtime	Night	Notes
Blood Sugar									
Insulin Dose									
Grams Carb									
Activity									

Date:	Breakfast	Snack	Lunch	Snack	Dinner	Snack	Bedtime	Night	Notes
Blood Sugar									
Insulin Dose									
Grams Carb									
Activity									

Date:	Breakfast	Snack	Lunch	Snack	Dinner	Snack	Bedtime	Night	Notes
Blood Sugar									
Insulin Dose									
Grams Carb									
Activity									

Date:	Breakfast	Snack	Lunch	Snack	Dinner	Snack	Bedtime	Night	Notes
Blood Sugar									
Insulin Dose									
Grams Carb									
Activity									

Weekly Diabetes Record

Name: _____

Date:	Breakfast	Snack	Lunch	Snack	Dinner	Snack	Bedtime	Night	Notes
Blood Sugar									
Insulin Dose									
Grams Carb									
Activity									

Date:	Breakfast	Snack	Lunch	Snack	Dinner	Snack	Bedtime	Night	Notes
Blood Sugar									
Insulin Dose									
Grams Carb									
Activity									

Date:	Breakfast	Snack	Lunch	Snack	Dinner	Snack	Bedtime	Night	Notes
Blood Sugar									
Insulin Dose									
Grams Carb									
Activity									

Date:	Breakfast	Snack	Lunch	Snack	Dinner	Snack	Bedtime	Night	Notes
Blood Sugar									
Insulin Dose									
Grams Carb									
Activity									

Date:	Breakfast	Snack	Lunch	Snack	Dinner	Snack	Bedtime	Night	Notes
Blood Sugar									
Insulin Dose									
Grams Carb									
Activity									

Date:	Breakfast	Snack	Lunch	Snack	Dinner	Snack	Bedtime	Night	Notes
Blood Sugar									
Insulin Dose									
Grams Carb									
Activity									

Date:	Breakfast	Snack	Lunch	Snack	Dinner	Snack	Bedtime	Night	Notes
Blood Sugar									
Insulin Dose									
Grams Carb									
Activity									

Weekly Diabetes Record

Name: _____

Date:	Breakfast	Snack	Lunch	Snack	Dinner	Snack	Bedtime	Night	Notes
Blood Sugar									
Insulin Dose									
Grams Carb									
Activity									

Date:	Breakfast	Snack	Lunch	Snack	Dinner	Snack	Bedtime	Night	Notes
Blood Sugar									
Insulin Dose									
Grams Carb									
Activity									

Date:	Breakfast	Snack	Lunch	Snack	Dinner	Snack	Bedtime	Night	Notes
Blood Sugar									
Insulin Dose									
Grams Carb									
Activity									

Date:	Breakfast	Snack	Lunch	Snack	Dinner	Snack	Bedtime	Night	Notes
Blood Sugar									
Insulin Dose									
Grams Carb									
Activity									

Date:	Breakfast	Snack	Lunch	Snack	Dinner	Snack	Bedtime	Night	Notes
Blood Sugar									
Insulin Dose									
Grams Carb									
Activity									

Date:	Breakfast	Snack	Lunch	Snack	Dinner	Snack	Bedtime	Night	Notes
Blood Sugar									
Insulin Dose									
Grams Carb									
Activity									

Date:	Breakfast	Snack	Lunch	Snack	Dinner	Snack	Bedtime	Night	Notes
Blood Sugar									
Insulin Dose									
Grams Carb									
Activity									

Weekly Diabetes Record

Name: _____

Date:	Breakfast	Snack	Lunch	Snack	Dinner	Snack	Bedtime	Night	Notes
Blood Sugar									
Insulin Dose									
Grams Carb									
Activity									

Date:	Breakfast	Snack	Lunch	Snack	Dinner	Snack	Bedtime	Night	Notes
Blood Sugar									
Insulin Dose									
Grams Carb									
Activity									

Date:	Breakfast	Snack	Lunch	Snack	Dinner	Snack	Bedtime	Night	Notes
Blood Sugar									
Insulin Dose									
Grams Carb									
Activity									

Date:	Breakfast	Snack	Lunch	Snack	Dinner	Snack	Bedtime	Night	Notes
Blood Sugar									
Insulin Dose									
Grams Carb									
Activity									

Date:	Breakfast	Snack	Lunch	Snack	Dinner	Snack	Bedtime	Night	Notes
Blood Sugar									
Insulin Dose									
Grams Carb									
Activity									

Date:	Breakfast	Snack	Lunch	Snack	Dinner	Snack	Bedtime	Night	Notes
Blood Sugar									
Insulin Dose									
Grams Carb									
Activity									

Date:	Breakfast	Snack	Lunch	Snack	Dinner	Snack	Bedtime	Night	Notes
Blood Sugar									
Insulin Dose									
Grams Carb									
Activity									

Weekly Diabetes Record

Name: _____

Date:	Breakfast	Snack	Lunch	Snack	Dinner	Snack	Bedtime	Night	Notes
Blood Sugar									
Insulin Dose									
Grams Carb									
Activity									

Date:	Breakfast	Snack	Lunch	Snack	Dinner	Snack	Bedtime	Night	Notes
Blood Sugar									
Insulin Dose									
Grams Carb									
Activity									

Date:	Breakfast	Snack	Lunch	Snack	Dinner	Snack	Bedtime	Night	Notes
Blood Sugar									
Insulin Dose									
Grams Carb									
Activity									

Date:	Breakfast	Snack	Lunch	Snack	Dinner	Snack	Bedtime	Night	Notes
Blood Sugar									
Insulin Dose									
Grams Carb									
Activity									

Date:	Breakfast	Snack	Lunch	Snack	Dinner	Snack	Bedtime	Night	Notes
Blood Sugar									
Insulin Dose									
Grams Carb									
Activity									

Date:	Breakfast	Snack	Lunch	Snack	Dinner	Snack	Bedtime	Night	Notes
Blood Sugar									
Insulin Dose									
Grams Carb									
Activity									

Date:	Breakfast	Snack	Lunch	Snack	Dinner	Snack	Bedtime	Night	Notes
Blood Sugar									
Insulin Dose									
Grams Carb									
Activity									

Weekly Diabetes Record

Name: _____

Date:	Breakfast	Snack	Lunch	Snack	Dinner	Snack	Bedtime	Night	Notes
Blood Sugar									
Insulin Dose									
Grams Carb									
Activity									

Date:	Breakfast	Snack	Lunch	Snack	Dinner	Snack	Bedtime	Night	Notes
Blood Sugar									
Insulin Dose									
Grams Carb									
Activity									

Date:	Breakfast	Snack	Lunch	Snack	Dinner	Snack	Bedtime	Night	Notes
Blood Sugar									
Insulin Dose									
Grams Carb									
Activity									

Date:	Breakfast	Snack	Lunch	Snack	Dinner	Snack	Bedtime	Night	Notes
Blood Sugar									
Insulin Dose									
Grams Carb									
Activity									

Date:	Breakfast	Snack	Lunch	Snack	Dinner	Snack	Bedtime	Night	Notes
Blood Sugar									
Insulin Dose									
Grams Carb									
Activity									

Date:	Breakfast	Snack	Lunch	Snack	Dinner	Snack	Bedtime	Night	Notes
Blood Sugar									
Insulin Dose									
Grams Carb									
Activity									

Date:	Breakfast	Snack	Lunch	Snack	Dinner	Snack	Bedtime	Night	Notes
Blood Sugar									
Insulin Dose									
Grams Carb									
Activity									

Weekly Diabetes Record

Name: _____

Date:	Breakfast	Snack	Lunch	Snack	Dinner	Snack	Bedtime	Night	Notes
Blood Sugar									
Insulin Dose									
Grams Carb									
Activity									

Date:	Breakfast	Snack	Lunch	Snack	Dinner	Snack	Bedtime	Night	Notes
Blood Sugar									
Insulin Dose									
Grams Carb									
Activity									

Date:	Breakfast	Snack	Lunch	Snack	Dinner	Snack	Bedtime	Night	Notes
Blood Sugar									
Insulin Dose									
Grams Carb									
Activity									

Date:	Breakfast	Snack	Lunch	Snack	Dinner	Snack	Bedtime	Night	Notes
Blood Sugar									
Insulin Dose									
Grams Carb									
Activity									

Date:	Breakfast	Snack	Lunch	Snack	Dinner	Snack	Bedtime	Night	Notes
Blood Sugar									
Insulin Dose									
Grams Carb									
Activity									

Date:	Breakfast	Snack	Lunch	Snack	Dinner	Snack	Bedtime	Night	Notes
Blood Sugar									
Insulin Dose									
Grams Carb									
Activity									

Date:	Breakfast	Snack	Lunch	Snack	Dinner	Snack	Bedtime	Night	Notes
Blood Sugar									
Insulin Dose									
Grams Carb									
Activity									

Weekly Diabetes Record

Name: _____

Date:	Breakfast	Snack	Lunch	Snack	Dinner	Snack	Bedtime	Night	Notes
Blood Sugar									
Insulin Dose									
Grams Carb									
Activity									

Date:	Breakfast	Snack	Lunch	Snack	Dinner	Snack	Bedtime	Night	Notes
Blood Sugar									
Insulin Dose									
Grams Carb									
Activity									

Date:	Breakfast	Snack	Lunch	Snack	Dinner	Snack	Bedtime	Night	Notes
Blood Sugar									
Insulin Dose									
Grams Carb									
Activity									

Date:	Breakfast	Snack	Lunch	Snack	Dinner	Snack	Bedtime	Night	Notes
Blood Sugar									
Insulin Dose									
Grams Carb									
Activity									

Date:	Breakfast	Snack	Lunch	Snack	Dinner	Snack	Bedtime	Night	Notes
Blood Sugar									
Insulin Dose									
Grams Carb									
Activity									

Date:	Breakfast	Snack	Lunch	Snack	Dinner	Snack	Bedtime	Night	Notes
Blood Sugar									
Insulin Dose									
Grams Carb									
Activity									

Date:	Breakfast	Snack	Lunch	Snack	Dinner	Snack	Bedtime	Night	Notes
Blood Sugar									
Insulin Dose									
Grams Carb									
Activity									

Weekly Diabetes Record

Name: _____

Date:	Breakfast	Snack	Lunch	Snack	Dinner	Snack	Bedtime	Night	Notes
Blood Sugar									
Insulin Dose									
Grams Carb									
Activity									

Date:	Breakfast	Snack	Lunch	Snack	Dinner	Snack	Bedtime	Night	Notes
Blood Sugar									
Insulin Dose									
Grams Carb									
Activity									

Date:	Breakfast	Snack	Lunch	Snack	Dinner	Snack	Bedtime	Night	Notes
Blood Sugar									
Insulin Dose									
Grams Carb									
Activity									

Date:	Breakfast	Snack	Lunch	Snack	Dinner	Snack	Bedtime	Night	Notes
Blood Sugar									
Insulin Dose									
Grams Carb									
Activity									

Date:	Breakfast	Snack	Lunch	Snack	Dinner	Snack	Bedtime	Night	Notes
Blood Sugar									
Insulin Dose									
Grams Carb									
Activity									

Date:	Breakfast	Snack	Lunch	Snack	Dinner	Snack	Bedtime	Night	Notes
Blood Sugar									
Insulin Dose									
Grams Carb									
Activity									

Date:	Breakfast	Snack	Lunch	Snack	Dinner	Snack	Bedtime	Night	Notes
Blood Sugar									
Insulin Dose									
Grams Carb									
Activity									

Weekly Diabetes Record

Name: _____

Date:	Breakfast	Snack	Lunch	Snack	Dinner	Snack	Bedtime	Night	Notes
Blood Sugar									
Insulin Dose									
Grams Carb									
Activity									

Date:	Breakfast	Snack	Lunch	Snack	Dinner	Snack	Bedtime	Night	Notes
Blood Sugar									
Insulin Dose									
Grams Carb									
Activity									

Date:	Breakfast	Snack	Lunch	Snack	Dinner	Snack	Bedtime	Night	Notes
Blood Sugar									
Insulin Dose									
Grams Carb									
Activity									

Date:	Breakfast	Snack	Lunch	Snack	Dinner	Snack	Bedtime	Night	Notes
Blood Sugar									
Insulin Dose									
Grams Carb									
Activity									

Date:	Breakfast	Snack	Lunch	Snack	Dinner	Snack	Bedtime	Night	Notes
Blood Sugar									
Insulin Dose									
Grams Carb									
Activity									

Date:	Breakfast	Snack	Lunch	Snack	Dinner	Snack	Bedtime	Night	Notes
Blood Sugar									
Insulin Dose									
Grams Carb									
Activity									

Date:	Breakfast	Snack	Lunch	Snack	Dinner	Snack	Bedtime	Night	Notes
Blood Sugar									
Insulin Dose									
Grams Carb									
Activity									

Weekly Diabetes Record

Name: _____

Date:	Breakfast	Snack	Lunch	Snack	Dinner	Snack	Bedtime	Night	Notes
Blood Sugar									
Insulin Dose									
Grams Carb									
Activity									

Date:	Breakfast	Snack	Lunch	Snack	Dinner	Snack	Bedtime	Night	Notes
Blood Sugar									
Insulin Dose									
Grams Carb									
Activity									

Date:	Breakfast	Snack	Lunch	Snack	Dinner	Snack	Bedtime	Night	Notes
Blood Sugar									
Insulin Dose									
Grams Carb									
Activity									

Date:	Breakfast	Snack	Lunch	Snack	Dinner	Snack	Bedtime	Night	Notes
Blood Sugar									
Insulin Dose									
Grams Carb									
Activity									

Date:	Breakfast	Snack	Lunch	Snack	Dinner	Snack	Bedtime	Night	Notes
Blood Sugar									
Insulin Dose									
Grams Carb									
Activity									

Date:	Breakfast	Snack	Lunch	Snack	Dinner	Snack	Bedtime	Night	Notes
Blood Sugar									
Insulin Dose									
Grams Carb									
Activity									

Date:	Breakfast	Snack	Lunch	Snack	Dinner	Snack	Bedtime	Night	Notes
Blood Sugar									
Insulin Dose									
Grams Carb									
Activity									

Weekly Diabetes Record

Name: _____

Date:	Breakfast	Snack	Lunch	Snack	Dinner	Snack	Bedtime	Night	Notes
Blood Sugar									
Insulin Dose									
Grams Carb									
Activity									

Date:	Breakfast	Snack	Lunch	Snack	Dinner	Snack	Bedtime	Night	Notes
Blood Sugar									
Insulin Dose									
Grams Carb									
Activity									

Date:	Breakfast	Snack	Lunch	Snack	Dinner	Snack	Bedtime	Night	Notes
Blood Sugar									
Insulin Dose									
Grams Carb									
Activity									

Date:	Breakfast	Snack	Lunch	Snack	Dinner	Snack	Bedtime	Night	Notes
Blood Sugar									
Insulin Dose									
Grams Carb									
Activity									

Date:	Breakfast	Snack	Lunch	Snack	Dinner	Snack	Bedtime	Night	Notes
Blood Sugar									
Insulin Dose									
Grams Carb									
Activity									

Date:	Breakfast	Snack	Lunch	Snack	Dinner	Snack	Bedtime	Night	Notes
Blood Sugar									
Insulin Dose									
Grams Carb									
Activity									

Date:	Breakfast	Snack	Lunch	Snack	Dinner	Snack	Bedtime	Night	Notes
Blood Sugar									
Insulin Dose									
Grams Carb									
Activity									

Weekly Diabetes Record

Name: _____

Date:	Breakfast	Snack	Lunch	Snack	Dinner	Snack	Bedtime	Night	Notes
Blood Sugar									
Insulin Dose									
Grams Carb									
Activity									

Date:	Breakfast	Snack	Lunch	Snack	Dinner	Snack	Bedtime	Night	Notes
Blood Sugar									
Insulin Dose									
Grams Carb									
Activity									

Date:	Breakfast	Snack	Lunch	Snack	Dinner	Snack	Bedtime	Night	Notes
Blood Sugar									
Insulin Dose									
Grams Carb									
Activity									

Date:	Breakfast	Snack	Lunch	Snack	Dinner	Snack	Bedtime	Night	Notes
Blood Sugar									
Insulin Dose									
Grams Carb									
Activity									

Date:	Breakfast	Snack	Lunch	Snack	Dinner	Snack	Bedtime	Night	Notes
Blood Sugar									
Insulin Dose									
Grams Carb									
Activity									

Date:	Breakfast	Snack	Lunch	Snack	Dinner	Snack	Bedtime	Night	Notes
Blood Sugar									
Insulin Dose									
Grams Carb									
Activity									

Date:	Breakfast	Snack	Lunch	Snack	Dinner	Snack	Bedtime	Night	Notes
Blood Sugar									
Insulin Dose									
Grams Carb									
Activity									

Weekly Diabetes Record

Name: _____

Date:	Breakfast	Snack	Lunch	Snack	Dinner	Snack	Bedtime	Night	Notes
Blood Sugar									
Insulin Dose									
Grams Carb									
Activity									

Date:	Breakfast	Snack	Lunch	Snack	Dinner	Snack	Bedtime	Night	Notes
Blood Sugar									
Insulin Dose									
Grams Carb									
Activity									

Date:	Breakfast	Snack	Lunch	Snack	Dinner	Snack	Bedtime	Night	Notes
Blood Sugar									
Insulin Dose									
Grams Carb									
Activity									

Date:	Breakfast	Snack	Lunch	Snack	Dinner	Snack	Bedtime	Night	Notes
Blood Sugar									
Insulin Dose									
Grams Carb									
Activity									

Date:	Breakfast	Snack	Lunch	Snack	Dinner	Snack	Bedtime	Night	Notes
Blood Sugar									
Insulin Dose									
Grams Carb									
Activity									

Date:	Breakfast	Snack	Lunch	Snack	Dinner	Snack	Bedtime	Night	Notes
Blood Sugar									
Insulin Dose									
Grams Carb									
Activity									

Date:	Breakfast	Snack	Lunch	Snack	Dinner	Snack	Bedtime	Night	Notes
Blood Sugar									
Insulin Dose									
Grams Carb									
Activity									

Weekly Diabetes Record

Name: _____

Date:	Breakfast	Snack	Lunch	Snack	Dinner	Snack	Bedtime	Night	Notes
Blood Sugar									
Insulin Dose									
Grams Carb									
Activity									

Date:	Breakfast	Snack	Lunch	Snack	Dinner	Snack	Bedtime	Night	Notes
Blood Sugar									
Insulin Dose									
Grams Carb									
Activity									

Date:	Breakfast	Snack	Lunch	Snack	Dinner	Snack	Bedtime	Night	Notes
Blood Sugar									
Insulin Dose									
Grams Carb									
Activity									

Date:	Breakfast	Snack	Lunch	Snack	Dinner	Snack	Bedtime	Night	Notes
Blood Sugar									
Insulin Dose									
Grams Carb									
Activity									

Date:	Breakfast	Snack	Lunch	Snack	Dinner	Snack	Bedtime	Night	Notes
Blood Sugar									
Insulin Dose									
Grams Carb									
Activity									

Date:	Breakfast	Snack	Lunch	Snack	Dinner	Snack	Bedtime	Night	Notes
Blood Sugar									
Insulin Dose									
Grams Carb									
Activity									

Date:	Breakfast	Snack	Lunch	Snack	Dinner	Snack	Bedtime	Night	Notes
Blood Sugar									
Insulin Dose									
Grams Carb									
Activity									

Weekly Diabetes Record

Name: _____

Date:	Breakfast	Snack	Lunch	Snack	Dinner	Snack	Bedtime	Night	Notes
Blood Sugar									
Insulin Dose									
Grams Carb									
Activity									

Date:	Breakfast	Snack	Lunch	Snack	Dinner	Snack	Bedtime	Night	Notes
Blood Sugar									
Insulin Dose									
Grams Carb									
Activity									

Date:	Breakfast	Snack	Lunch	Snack	Dinner	Snack	Bedtime	Night	Notes
Blood Sugar									
Insulin Dose									
Grams Carb									
Activity									

Date:	Breakfast	Snack	Lunch	Snack	Dinner	Snack	Bedtime	Night	Notes
Blood Sugar									
Insulin Dose									
Grams Carb									
Activity									

Date:	Breakfast	Snack	Lunch	Snack	Dinner	Snack	Bedtime	Night	Notes
Blood Sugar									
Insulin Dose									
Grams Carb									
Activity									

Date:	Breakfast	Snack	Lunch	Snack	Dinner	Snack	Bedtime	Night	Notes
Blood Sugar									
Insulin Dose									
Grams Carb									
Activity									

Date:	Breakfast	Snack	Lunch	Snack	Dinner	Snack	Bedtime	Night	Notes
Blood Sugar									
Insulin Dose									
Grams Carb									
Activity									

Weekly Diabetes Record

Name: _____

Date:	Breakfast	Snack	Lunch	Snack	Dinner	Snack	Bedtime	Night	Notes
Blood Sugar									
Insulin Dose									
Grams Carb									
Activity									

Date:	Breakfast	Snack	Lunch	Snack	Dinner	Snack	Bedtime	Night	Notes
Blood Sugar									
Insulin Dose									
Grams Carb									
Activity									

Date:	Breakfast	Snack	Lunch	Snack	Dinner	Snack	Bedtime	Night	Notes
Blood Sugar									
Insulin Dose									
Grams Carb									
Activity									

Date:	Breakfast	Snack	Lunch	Snack	Dinner	Snack	Bedtime	Night	Notes
Blood Sugar									
Insulin Dose									
Grams Carb									
Activity									

Date:	Breakfast	Snack	Lunch	Snack	Dinner	Snack	Bedtime	Night	Notes
Blood Sugar									
Insulin Dose									
Grams Carb									
Activity									

Date:	Breakfast	Snack	Lunch	Snack	Dinner	Snack	Bedtime	Night	Notes
Blood Sugar									
Insulin Dose									
Grams Carb									
Activity									

Date:	Breakfast	Snack	Lunch	Snack	Dinner	Snack	Bedtime	Night	Notes
Blood Sugar									
Insulin Dose									
Grams Carb									
Activity									

Weekly Diabetes Record

Name: _____

Date:	Breakfast	Snack	Lunch	Snack	Dinner	Snack	Bedtime	Night	Notes
Blood Sugar									
Insulin Dose									
Grams Carb									
Activity									

Date:	Breakfast	Snack	Lunch	Snack	Dinner	Snack	Bedtime	Night	Notes
Blood Sugar									
Insulin Dose									
Grams Carb									
Activity									

Date:	Breakfast	Snack	Lunch	Snack	Dinner	Snack	Bedtime	Night	Notes
Blood Sugar									
Insulin Dose									
Grams Carb									
Activity									

Date:	Breakfast	Snack	Lunch	Snack	Dinner	Snack	Bedtime	Night	Notes
Blood Sugar									
Insulin Dose									
Grams Carb									
Activity									

Date:	Breakfast	Snack	Lunch	Snack	Dinner	Snack	Bedtime	Night	Notes
Blood Sugar									
Insulin Dose									
Grams Carb									
Activity									

Date:	Breakfast	Snack	Lunch	Snack	Dinner	Snack	Bedtime	Night	Notes
Blood Sugar									
Insulin Dose									
Grams Carb									
Activity									

Date:	Breakfast	Snack	Lunch	Snack	Dinner	Snack	Bedtime	Night	Notes
Blood Sugar									
Insulin Dose									
Grams Carb									
Activity